Sex and Your Teenager

A Parent's Guide

John Coleman

Trust for the Study of Adolescence, Brighton

JOHN WILEY & SONS, LTD

Chichester · New York · Weinheim · Brisbane · Singapore · Toronto

Copyright © 2001 by   John Wiley & Sons Ltd,
                      Baffins Lane, Chichester,
                      West Sussex PO19 1UD, England

                      National   01243 779777
                      International (+44) 1243 779777
                      e-mail (for orders and customer service enquiries):
                      cs-books@wiley.co.uk
                      Visit our Home Page on http://www.wiley.co.uk
                                          or http://www.wiley.com

Other Wiley Editorial Offices

John Wiley & Sons, Inc., 605 Third Avenue,
New York, NY 10158-0012, USA

WILEY-VCH GmbH, Pappelallee 3,
D-69469 Weinheim, Germany

John Wiley & Sons Australia, Ltd, 33 Park Road, Milton,
Queensland 4064, Australia

John Wiley & Sons (Asia) Pte Ltd, 2 Clementi Loop #02-01,
Jin Xing Distripark, Singapore 129809

John Wiley & Sons (Canada) Ltd, 22 Worcester Road,
Rexdale, Ontario M9W 1L1, Canada

British Library Cataloguing in Publication Data
A catalogue record for this book is available from the British Library

ISBN 0-471-48562-4

Project management by Originator, Gt Yarmouth, Norfolk (typeset in 11.5/13 Imprint)
Printed and bound in Great Britain by Biddles Ltd, Guildford and King's Lynn
This book is printed on acid-free paper responsibly manufactured from sustainable
forestry, in which at least two trees are planted for each one used for paper production.

Contents

About the author

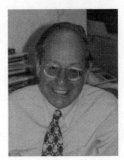

Dr John Coleman trained as a clinical psychologist at the Middlesex Hospital, London. He worked for 14 years as a Senior Lecturer in the Department of Psychiatry at the Royal London Hospital. Since 1988 he has been the Director of the Trust for the Study of Adolescence, an independent research and training organisation based in Brighton. He has written widely on the subject of adolescence, including *Key Data on Adolescence* (2001) and *The Nature of Adolescence* (1999). In 2001 he was awarded the OBE for services to youth justice.

Foreword

When you talk to adults about the sex education they received, they will generally say that it was totally inadequate and that they want something better for their children. So it is not surprising that research shows that parents think that they should talk to their children about sex and relationships. In addition, contrary to common belief, children want this dialogue with their parent too. But even today, when there is so much discussion of sex around us, the reality of family communication rarely meets the aspirations of parents or children.

Sex and Your Teenager is a valuable tool to help fill this gap. It provides clear information and practical, down-to-earth advice to assist parents in supporting their children as they grow into adulthood. John Coleman's own commitment to improving the lives of young people and their families and his comprehensive expertise shine through his inspirational book. I am sure that any parent who reads it will find their knowledge increased and their confidence enhanced. As a result, they will find it easier to communicate with their children about sex and relationships, to give them the understanding and confidence to establish fulfilling and rewarding relationships in the future.

Anne Weyman, OBE
Chief Executive
Family Planning Association

Introduction

This is a book for parents and all who care for young people. There are many books, pamphlets, leaflets and so on available for teenagers, but there are few books which are written for mothers and fathers, step-parents, foster parents and other carers. In the chapters that follow, I will cover some of the issues that I believe are of concern to adults. Sexuality is not an easy topic for parents and carers to deal with once their children enter adolescence. Everyone is aware of the need to discuss sex with a teenager. The only question is: How to start the conversation? The experience of this mother and daughter will be familiar to countless adults who have struggled with this problem:

And one day I remember I was walking along the track, and Mum says to me 'So you know how to do it now then?' So I said 'Well I knew already, like, you know, because I did.' Then she said 'You know properly now and all this lot.' And I was

*getting really embarrassed and I was saying 'yeh',
like this, and I was trying to get on to a different
subject. And she was saying 'So you know how to
make a baby and how to look after a baby' and all
this rubbish. So I goes 'Yes, Mum' and I was
trying to get off the subject all the time.*

There is no doubt that the first and overwhelming
obstacle is embarrassment. Many adults put this down
to the poor sex education they themselves received. This
may be a factor, but other things play their part. Sexuality
causes all sorts of complex feelings within a family, and
these feelings have the effect of creating taboos and
inhibitions. We will be looking at some of these in the
course of this book.

In addition to embarrassment, parents face other
difficulties when it comes to dealing with teenage sexuality. Some feel inadequate – uncertain what to say or how
to cope with conflicts over values and attitudes. Others
find themselves getting anxious about what is going on
in sex-education lessons at school, or the possibility of
an unwanted pregnancy. Such worries may lead them to
behave in a fussy or overprotective fashion. On top of all
this, there are parents who feel quite simply out of their
depth. The very idea of talking about sex and sexuality
may be something which is quite foreign to them. They
realise that their son or daughter is growing up, they know
that parents ought to say something, but they are unable
to do anything about it.

I hope that all parents and carers, whether shy or
anxious, confident or embarrassed, will find something
of value in this book.

Puberty

Puberty is the point in a young person's development when the body begins to change from that of a child to that of an adult. Puberty is not one single event, but many different events, and it takes place over quite a long period of time – usually about two years.

Of course, sexuality does not begin with puberty. There are many ways in which children make it clear that they are sexual beings. They are curious about their own bodies. They ask questions about their parents' bodies. They may masturbate, or find other ways of giving themselves bodily comfort or pleasure. They are aware of gender differences. All these are reflections of the fact that sexuality develops gradually from infancy onwards. When puberty arrives, your child will not be a complete stranger to thoughts and ideas of a sexual nature.

Puberty is, however, a critical moment in the overall process of growing up. It is during this stage that your child's body develops the characteristics of a sexually mature adult. In addition, a wide range of emotional and psychological changes begin to take place. All of these are

part of the essential preparation for adulthood in which
every teenager is involved.

In this chapter, I will cover:

Bodily changes in girls

Bodily changes in boys

The age of puberty

The emotional consequences of puberty

Periods

Wet dreams

Whether puberty is starting earlier than in
previous generations

Bodily changes in girls

The whole process of puberty is thought to take about two
years, although in some cases it may take longer. During
this time many different changes occur in the body. For
girls the most important of these are:

- the growth spurt (when girls start to grow taller and
  heavier);
- the development of sexual organs, such as the uterus
  and the vagina;
- the growth of the heart, the lungs and other major
  organs of the body;
- changes in the composition of the blood and in
  hormone levels;

- the development of the breasts and the hips;
- the growth of hair on the body – in particular under the arms and around the pubic area;
- the start of menstruation.

When the changes are listed in this way, you can see how puberty affects almost every aspect of bodily functioning. Obviously the changes do not all occur at the same time. For girls, the appearance of pubic hair or the beginnings of breast development are most likely to signal the start of puberty.

Periods are likely to begin fairly late in the sequence, after hormone levels have altered and internal sexual organs have matured.

Bodily changes in boys

Boys too experience many bodily changes during puberty. The most important of these are:

- the growth spurt (when boys start to grow taller and heavier, and to develop a more muscular body);
- the development of the sexual organs such as the penis and the testicles;
- changes in the composition of the blood and in hormone levels;
- the growth of the lungs, the heart and other major organs of the body;
- the breaking of the voice;
- the growth of hair on the body – in particular, on the face, under the arms and in the pubic region;
- the start of wet dreams (when the boy becomes sexually aroused during sleep, and his penis emits semen).

As with girls these changes are very far-reaching, and affect all parts of the body. While no two boys progress through puberty in exactly the same way, for most the beginning of the growth spurt indicates the start of puberty, while wet dreams usually occur towards the end of the sequence. Wet dreams indicate that the boy has now become sexually mature.

The age of puberty

In recent years, there has been a lot of debate about the age of puberty. Many believe it is beginning earlier and earlier, while others think this is a myth. I will deal with this controversial question in a section at the end of the chapter. First, I wish to consider some general issues concerning the age of puberty.

The first thing to say is that boys and girls differ in the age at which they reach puberty. Boys are usually about 18 months to two years behind girls. On average, in Western industrialised countries, girls start puberty between 10 and 11, while boys start between 11 and 12. These figures, are of course, only an average, and it is important to remember that there is enormous individual variation. Imagine a picture of three 13-year-old girls. One is physically still a child, with no breast development and no pubic hair. Another is just in the middle of puberty, with budding breasts and pubic hair starting to show. The third girl is completely mature – she has a woman's body, her periods have started and she is fully developed in all areas. The three girls may at this stage feel very different. They look different, their friendships and interests may be different. However, in a few years the first two will have caught up with the third, and their differing rates of development will no longer mean very much to them.

There are a few young people – and it is only a small number – who may be classified as late developers. They are two or more years behind the majority in reaching puberty. As far as we know, except in extreme cases, this has no effect on them as adults. Yet, it may make social life difficult for a while. Adults need to be sensitive to the needs of these particular boys and girls. They may well require a bit of extra support, as well as reassurance that they will catch up in due course.

At the opposite end of the spectrum, some children develop much earlier than the average:

> *Well, I think I probably physically changed a lot younger than all my schoolmates. And that was very embarrassing in a sort of middle-school environment. Where, you know, if I was wearing a bra all the boys would go round pinging at me, just being thoroughly annoying. And that was very embarrassing. But with the help of my parents, 'cos I would go home and discuss it with them ... They'd say you must understand that they're not going through that and they don't know that, and you'll have to bear with it for the moment. After that, I think I coped with it very well. But it was difficult at first.*
>
> 16-year-old girl

Most boys who develop early seem to be at an advantage, since their strength and athletic skills make them popular with the crowd. For early-developing girls, the picture is more mixed. Such girls may be socially popular with older boys, but they may be resented by other girls. This may lead to them being excluded from female activities. Also, their physical maturity may not be matched by their emotional maturity. Girls who reach puberty very early may also need some extra support from adults.

The emotional consequences of puberty

Clearly, such major bodily changes cannot occur without their being very important psychological consequences. Your child may be unsettled by the changes to his or her body. He or she may feel odd, or feel different. Young people may sometimes even find that they don't recognise themselves in the mirror.

After all, it takes time to come to terms with increased size, new muscles, a strange body. This may well lead to a stage of clumsiness and awkwardness. All this together, combined with the physical changes, can make your teenager extremely self-conscious.

Young people experience a range of new feelings as a result of hormonal changes. Some of these may be good feelings, but there will also be more moodiness and depression. Adults should not be surprised if, during this stage, teenagers appear to be more affected by their emotions than when they were younger. They may well swing sharply from one mood to another. All this is quite normal – part of the process of adjusting to the changes of puberty.

Girls and boys at this age are more prone to doubts and uncertainties about themselves. The changing body leads to a changing sense of self, and may well lead to a number of anxieties. Some of these will have to do with physical concerns. Am I normal? Is my body the right shape? How can I cure my spots? Am I overweight? Are my breasts too big? Is my penis too small?

I remember my daughter saying 'I've got these lumps, I've got these lumps', you know, and it was like 'oh well, don't worry, you know, it's breasts starting to grow'. And then it was 'but it hurts', so then you find out that that's quite normal, and they don't always grow at the same rate, and she's reassured. I think we went through quite a few phases of things not being unexpected, but not being quite how you might have expected them to be, not necessarily all that straight-forward and sort of minor panics. Usually I would say 'don't worry I am sure it is perfectly normal', but at the same time you know they're bound to worry.

Mother of one daughter and two sons

Other worries have more to do with social issues about friends, about dating, about the sort of person the girl or boy is, or is going to become. Again, concerns at this age are important elements of the process of growing up. They are a necessary part of your teenager changing from a child to an adult.

Periods

Since this is a book for adults rather than for young people, I will not go into great detail about periods, and how they start. There are many useful books for teenagers on this subject, and it is certainly a good idea for every family to have one or two around. You will find some suggestions at the end of the chapter.

What sort of problems do parents and carers face when thinking about a girl's first period? The most obvious issue has to do with preparation. However determined

you are to make sure that the young person is well prepared, in the event it won't necessarily be easy. You may
find it embarrassing to talk about – more embarrassing
than either of you expects. Or it may be hard to find the
right time. When the girl is nine years old may seem too
early, but at ten it may be too late. Also, it has to be said
that some children are more open and curious than others.
One girl may be chatty and perfectly relaxed about subjects to do with her body, and may like talking intimately
with her mother or a close adult. Another girl – even in the
same family – may be shy and awkward when it comes to
talking about personal matters.

Parents and carers should make sure that the girl is
properly prepared and well informed about menstruation.
The best time to do this is probably just at the point when
puberty is beginning. As we have noted, each girl is
different, so there is no general rule about the correct
age. Parents need to be aware of the girl's development,
and when the first signs of puberty become obvious (such
as changes in the girl's breasts) this is the time to start
talking about periods. This is also the time you need to
think about buying the first bra (a training bra).

It is important to remember that a girl may be more
worried or frightened about the idea of periods than she
can express. The thought of losing blood can cause all
sorts of fears – both rational and irrational. These may
be difficult to share with anyone, even in the most
caring and supportive family. In interviews with teenagers, this is a theme which recurs time and time again:

*I remember my first fear, and hating it so much. I
thought I really don't want to go through this like, for
so many years. And I hated that, I really did. I sat
there and screamed and did just not want it at all. It
wasn't that I hadn't been prepared for it, I mean, I*

knew it was going to happen and everything. But I hadn't really prepared for what I was going to feel, the sort of feeling that I've got to go through this every month, blah, blah, blah, blah, and my mum just sort of said, yeh, look on it as a gift rather than you know, sort of like torture. But I mean to some extent you sort of think, I hate going through this every month.

15-year-old girl

However well prepared a girl is, there will always be some anxiety or embarrassment associated with the beginning of menstruation. So it is worthwhile to make sure that the girl has easy access to a suitable book or leaflet, in addition to talking about periods. This means that she can seek information at her own pace and in her own way. She may have practical questions which seem too silly to ask anyone about, or she may be fearful about something which is too embarrassing to express:

I mean I can remember the first day I learnt about periods from my friend. I was saying oh no, you know, I was terrified. I couldn't believe it, and I went home and asked my mum and she told me it was true. And I expected my mum to say no, no it's not true, and I was terrified.

14-year-old girl

Not all girls will be living with their own mother. Some may be cared for by fathers, stepmothers, foster mothers or other carers. In such circumstances, it may be even more difficult for the teenager to ask difficult questions, or share intimate worries and concerns. It is all the more important, therefore, for carers to ensure that girls know where to go for the information they need.

Wet dreams

A wet dream happens when a boy becomes sexually aroused during sleep to the point that he ejaculates (his penis emits semen). The first wet dream does not generally have the same degree of significance for a boy as the start of periods for a girl. Nonetheless, you should not underestimate the importance of wet dreams. They can cause a lot of anxiety, if the teenager is not properly prepared. The result of a wet dream, such as stains on the sheet, can be acutely embarrassing:

> *My youngest son, when he had a wet dream he was terribly embarrassed. Because he was actually going away to my sister's for the weekend, and I wanted him to take his duvet with him. And he said 'I can't, because it's got lions all over it' or something like that. I said for goodness sake it was your brother's before it was yours. And he looked so embarrassed. And I realised that he'd had a wet dream all over it, so I had to treat it terribly casually.*
>
> Mother of three sons

Sensitivity on the part of parents or carers is essential. In addition, it is obviously important for all boys to be properly prepared. While you don't need to make a big issue of it, simple information, such as the fact that almost all boys have wet dreams during puberty, will be reassuring.

Is puberty starting earlier than in previous generations?

As I have said, there has been much debate on this question in recent years. There is good evidence to show that in the first half of the 20th century the age of puberty in Western countries dropped substantially. It is thought that this was the result of better health care and improved nutrition. However, there is less certainty about what has been happening since the 1960s.

While some believe that the start of puberty continues to get younger and younger, others say that there is no good scientific evidence to support this belief. By and large, most teachers take the view that puberty is starting earlier, and that more girls are starting their periods in primary school than was the case 20 or 30 years ago. However, most doctors argue that, as yet, we do not have the research to support this claim.

What is fairly certain is that social behaviour has changed, with children of nine, ten or eleven getting involved in what were considered to be adolescent activities. Anyone watching a primary-school playground today will see how grown up many of the older children – the girls particularly – appear to be. This mature social behaviour may affect how we look at the 'pre-teen' age group, and may influence our beliefs about the age at which puberty is occurring.

Leaving this controversy on one side, we know that today a considerable number of girls are starting their periods before they reach secondary school. This is no longer an unusual happening, and should not cause any anxiety to you or to the girl herself. If this is the case with your daughter, you need to talk about it with the teacher. You need to ensure:

- that the school has proper facilities for the disposal of sanitary towels;
- that there is privacy for girls in the toilet area;
- that the school has an appropriate sex-education policy.

Both boys and girls need to know something about puberty and menstruation in primary school. By the time they reach secondary school, it is too late.

Conclusion

For the great majority of young people, puberty is a natural part of growing up. Many go through it without thinking very much about it – it is just something that happens. As one 15-year-old boy said when asked what he remembered about puberty, 'I hardly noticed it.' Nonetheless, there are some for whom puberty is a worry. This could be because:

- it comes very early;
- it comes very late;
- it causes anxieties and fears for which the young person is not prepared;
- the young person is especially self-conscious.

Let me take each of these in turn. First, those girls who start puberty early will develop breasts and start their periods before the rest of the peer group. These girls will be out of step with the majority, and may experience embarrassment and awkwardness. It may make friend-ships with other girls more dificult. It will certainly mean that boys will pay extra attention to these girls, making them stand out even more from the group. Parents, teachers and other adults do need to be aware of the problems that may arise for these early-maturing girls.

Second, there will be some, both boys and girls, who reach puberty much later than their peers. These young people also feel out of step. They may be excluded from social activities, and they may even be bullied. They will probably have all sorts of worries about the reasons for their late development, and what it means for their future. Consideration, understanding and support from adults are essential for these teenagers.

Third, there are those who have not been adequately prepared for puberty. Adolescents in this group are not always easy to spot. However, it is worth noting that preparation for puberty is never the responsibility of one adult alone. A teacher may be able to provide extra help for a pupil whose family has been disrupted by death or divorce. An aunt or older cousin may be able to offer information to a young person in a situation where the parent is unable to do so. Teenagers should not have to depend on one adult for all the support and information they need.

Lastly, a young person may be particularly self-conscious. This can mean that wearing a bra, or having to undress in a changing room after games, or being shorter than all your friends, causes acute embarrassment. There may not be a lot that adults can do. Nonetheless, sensitivity and understanding in the family can make all the difference to a young person whose changing body is causing distress.

For parents, too, puberty may not be much of a problem. Many find issues at this time easier to deal with than those that crop up at a later stage of adolescence. However, the problems I have just outlined for teenagers

can and do lead to difficulties in the home. It is important
to recognise, therefore, that puberty is not always easy for
parents. Difficulties may arise because of a deterioration
in communication, or because of marked changes in mood
or behaviour. Such changes may seem strange or worrying
to parents. Remember that there are likely to be good
reasons for the altered behaviour. These are addressed
in other chapters in this book, where you will also find
suggestions for further reading.

To conclude, here are some of the main facts about
puberty:

- it is a process that takes place over a period of time;
- it involves changes to the whole body, not just to the
  sexual organs;
- there is wide variation between individuals in the
  timing of puberty;
- girls reach puberty earlier than boys;
- with puberty comes a whole range of new feelings and
  emotions;
- the changes of puberty can lead to worries and anxieties.

The more information and preparation the young
person has, the better.

Useful reading

What Do You Want to Know about Puberty? by P.
Sanders and S. Myers – Franklin Watts (2000).

Everything You Ever Wanted to Ask About Periods
by Tricia Kreitman, Fiona Finlay and Rosemary
Jones – Piccadilly Press (2001). This includes

information on the biological and hormonal changes, as well as more practical tips.

What's Happening to My Body? A Growing-up Guide by Lynda Madaras – Penguin (1989). This book covers in detail the physical and emotional upheavals of puberty.

Useful websites

www.teenagehealthfreak.org a website for teenagers full of evidence-based medical information about common teenage health worries. Written by two doctors – Ann McPherson and Aidan Macfarlane.

2

Learning about sex

It is probably true to say that we learn about sex from the moment of birth. The fact is that the intimacy and nurturing involved in the mother–baby relationship creates a foundation stone for later sexuality. More broadly, however, the child learns about sex from school, from parents, from brothers, sisters, aunts, uncles, cousins and other relatives, from friends and neighbours, from the media, from books and films, from advertising, and from a host of other sources.

As I say, I was really young when I first began learning about sex. You sort of pick up words from school, and I think I got a rough idea from friends. You see people kissing on TV, and you think, well, that must have something to do with it. I didn't really know much about sex at all, and then when I saw it in textbooks and stuff like that it became clear. I couldn't say there was ever a time when I just suddenly knew it all, like, when I was 12, say. It was sort of a gradual

*kind of picking it up on the way. Nobody ever sat
down and told me. When I heard my friends talking
I sort of said, oh yeah, I know that, you know what I
mean? You're dying for them to say more, to see if you
can hear more and get a fair idea. You sort of push
them to say more so you pick up bits like that. It was
just a gradual process really that I learnt about sex. I
just didn't sort of like learn it in a day or whatever.*

                                            17-year-old girl

Children are curious about sex. After all, it is a fascinating
topic. Children are aware of much more that is going on
around them than adults realise and, of all the subjects
that children pay attention to, sex is probably top of the
list. When I talk about sex in this context, I do not refer
specifically to sexual intercourse. Sex is to do with love
and relationships, and this includes babies and where they
come from, differences between men and women, nudity,
kissing, what genitals are for and much else besides. All
these things are part of a large picture, and, throughout
childhood and adolescence, boys and girls are trying to
piece together what it all means. Children learn about
sex from many sources.

In this chapter, I will be considering the following topics:

                                Schools

                                Parents

                                Society

                                Friends

                            The media

                        Communication

Schools

In secondary schools, contraception and reproduction form part of National Curriculum Science and schools must deliver this. In addition, there is a legal requirement in schools to provide, as a minimum, information about sexually transmitted infections including HIV. Other aspects of sex education such as relationships, practising communication and negotiation skills and thinking about attitudes and beliefs are non-statutory and vary greatly from school to school. In July 2000, the government issued new guidelines on sex and relationship education, enshrined in legislation as part of the Learning and Skills Act (2000). This guidance states that such teaching (i.e. all teaching considered to cover non-biological aspects of sex) should be firmly rooted in Personal, Social, and Health Education (known as PSHE), and should be taught alongside the National Curriculum. All state secondary schools must have a policy on sex education, and this must be available to parents. Primary schools may decide themselves whether to provide sex education or not. Parents have the right to withdraw their children from any sex education lessons that do not form part of the National Curriculum.

It is a regrettable fact that, however determined a school is to provide high-quality sex education, there are numerous obstacles to be overcome. In the first place, the very distinction between biological and non-biological aspects of sex is unclear, and is bound to lead to confusion among pupils and teachers.

Second, over the last 20 years there has been an erosion of support for teachers wishing to teach this subject. Local education authorities have been forced to cut back on the numbers of health and sex-education advisors, thus reducing the amount of training and assistance available to teachers.

Other bodies, such as the Health Development Agency (formerly the Health Education Authority) have had their sphere of operations severely curtailed. In general, the climate within education is not conducive or supportive to the development of innovative approaches to sex education. In spite of this, there are examples of outstanding work being done in this area. Your child may be lucky enough to attend a school doing such work. Its excellence will almost certainly prove to be the result of the commitment and interest of individual teachers, however, rather than of policy within the education system.

Another problem faced by teachers is the enormous pressure on curriculum time. As examination results and league tables assume ever greater importance, inevitably non-examination subjects sink to the bottom of the priority list. Perhaps the time has come to rethink these priorities. After all, which is the more important – geography or sexuality? In my view, knowing about sexuality is going to have far more of a long-term impact in a child's life than being proficient in geography. What do you think?

A further difficulty for those involved in sex and relationships education has to do with morality and values. Indeed, much of the political debate has centred around the question of whether sex education should be taught within a 'moral' framework or not. Many argue that sexuality should be taught in the context of ideas about marriage and the family, and often in association with religious beliefs. Others, however, feel that this only alienates young people who may not share the religious views or moral attitudes of their teachers. It is this debate which creates so many of the obstacles hindering the development of high-quality education. It should be noted that Britain is not alone here. Similar, possibly worse, problems exist in the United States and in some other European countries, such as Italy and Spain. Yet Holland, Sweden and Denmark have managed to pioneer open and worthwhile programmes, and we have much to learn from these countries.

Families from minority ethnic cultures face particular problems here. They may find that their beliefs about sexuality are very different from those of the mainstream culture. This can cause conflict, and lead to difficulties between parents, school governors and education authorities. Just as in religious education, there needs to be recognition of the many faiths currently existing in Britain, so in sex education it is essential for schools to acknowledge that there will be different views about sex. Teenagers who are Asian, or Afro-Caribbean, or from countries such as the Sudan or Cyprus, may find themselves caught between the values of their friends, and those of their family. Schools have a critical role to play here in allowing young people to explore these differences. In addition, in the best of circumstances, schools can also help parents from all cultures to learn more about teenagers and sexuality.

Parents

It is very easy for parents to persuade themselves that their child's school is dealing with the tricky and embarrassing issue of sex education. This may let them off the hook, but, as I have just indicated, schools vary enormously in what they provide. Parents should not take refuge in the comforting thought that 'someone else is doing it'. Parents have responsibilities in relation to sex

education. Indeed, in the best circumstances the school
and the home should work in partnership, each providing
different elements of education for sexuality in the widest
sense:

> *I like sex education to start at school initially. We've*
> *been fortunate in that it has been done really for all*
> *my family. I like that because it starts them asking*
> *questions and then it's easier for you to go on from*
> *that. My own experience as a child was that my*
> *parents thought they'd taught me everything, and*
> *they'd taught me nothing at all. So I had a very*
> *confused idea about the whole thing. And my children*
> *are all much clearer in the head, and even my 12-*
> *year-old knows how periods are. I mean she has*
> *anxiety about it, but she has at least got some*
> *concept of that and also sexual relationships. I*
> *don't suppose she understands the emotional side of*
> *it yet, but again she has some idea at least, which is*
> *much easier to build on. That came from the school*
> *really.*

Mother of three daughters

As far as the school is concerned, the parents' responsibilities fall into three main areas. In the first place, it is up
to the parents to find out what is being taught. Parents
need to know which subjects are being covered, and at
what ages. Perhaps most importantly, they need to know
what their son or daughter thinks of the material. Did the
teenager still have unanswered questions? Were some
topics avoided, or presented too briefly? Were there
things the young person disagreed with? As we have
noted, the school should provide parents with information
about the sex education that is being taught, and parents
should be able to make use of this information.

Parents need to know what is going on in school:

- so that they can pick up on issues that are not covered;
- so that they can expand on things that are not clear;
- so that they can use the school's material as a spring-board for open discussion in the home.

There is another reason for parents to keep in close touch with what is being taught in school. Research shows clearly that the more interest and concern parents show in schoolwork, the better the young person's performance. Children and teenagers are very sensitive indeed to the way in which their parents value what they do. If parents take school seriously, and demonstrate this by asking questions and wanting to be informed, two messages come across clearly:

- 'I consider this to be important';
- 'I am interested in you, and in what you are doing'.

Lastly, it is worth noting that there are aspects of sexuality which the school simply cannot cover. The majority of sex education in school is likely to be factual, and to deal more often with the biology of sex than with the emotional and relationship side of things. Yet, we know from research that young people want opportunities to discuss the more personal aspects of sex – the tricky dilemmas of managing relationships and making choices about how to behave. Ideally, these should be dealt with at home as well as at school. In addition, with so many pupils in secondary schools it is difficult for teachers to take a personal interest in any one individual.

Most schools do have tutor schemes, or some form of support for each young person, but parents should never assume that this will meet all the teenager's needs. Young people need to know that there is someone who has a special concern for their welfare. That is the responsibility of parents or carers.

Society

The second half of the 20th century saw a revolution in sexual attitudes and behaviour. While this is not the place to enter into an extended discussion about the reasons for these historical changes, it is important to note some of the effects, especially those that have affected young people.

The first thing to look at is the contraceptive pill. The pill has, since the late 1960s, been available to any woman who wants it. This fact has resulted in the separation of sexual behaviour from procreation, for the first time in history. The impact of this cannot be overestimated.

Initially, the effect was felt by married women, who became able to control the timing of their pregnancies, and plan childbirth in a way that had never been possible before. In due course, however, more widespread effects became apparent. Men and women experienced greater sexual freedom, both within marriage and outside it. Not surprisingly, the possibilities of sexual experimentation were not lost on the young. It was this new-found freedom which, in part, led to the now famous – or infamous – permissiveness of the 1960s.

Another change has had to do with the public acceptability of sexual material. Today, no film is complete without an erotic, usually explicit, love scene. Much advertising depends on the use of sexual imagery. TV soaps compete to include sexual violence, underage sex, and so on. Teenage magazines appear to cover nothing but sexual matters. The f-word, once unacceptable in the paperback version of *Lady Chatterley's Lover*, is now so commonplace as to be hardly noticeable.

It is said that we live in an 'eroticised' society, where sex is everywhere. It is even said that there are no taboos left where sex is concerned, whereas we shall see that this is not the case. What is certainly true, however, is that the social changes that have occurred since the 1960s have had far-reaching effects on young people's lives.

The most obvious consequence for teenagers is that they cannot get away from sex. It is pervasive. Adults, who are more mature, may have better defences. They may be able to filter out what they don't want to hear. They may also have better control over their response to sexual messages. For teenagers, who have less maturity, less sexual experience and higher levels of anxiety about sexual matters anyway, this is not so easy. Although this is something that is rarely discussed, it should be a matter of concern. The fact that there is so much sex on public display is bound to create greater sexual arousal. Are we providing young people with the skills and resources to cope with this? I suspect not.

As a result of all this, it is not surprising to find that teenagers feel themselves under pressure to become sexually active. It is all too easy to gain the impression that 'everyone is doing it'. From this, it is but a simple step to the belief that, if everyone else is doing it, and you are not, then there must be something wrong with you. Pressures upon young people stem from friends, and from the wider peer group. These pressures may be quite open and direct. However, there is also a range of subtle and indirect pressures, including those created by the media and by the values of our culture. One of these values has to do with the right to expect sexual gratification. How could young people not be influenced by such an expectation?

A friend of mine did it with a boy when she was 13. She said 'Oh, you must, you must'. I listened because I was very influenced by other people, and she was my best friend and I had to do what she said or I wasn't in with her. I used to make it up that I did, but I didn't. So I didn't until I was 16, which was still quite young, but just so that I could be in with my friends.
                                                     18-year-old girl

There has been an unhealthy tendency among some groups of adults to blame the young for what is called 'sexual permissiveness'. Such a tendency is both short-sighted and hypocritical. The young do not set trends, they follow them. Teenagers are influenced in their behaviour primarily by what they see around them. Where sexuality is concerned, they learn from parents, and from neighbours. They learn from aunts and uncles, teachers and politicians – in short, they learn from adults. I call this 'invisible learning', because it does not involve lessons and textbooks. Neither does it involve any direct instruction or guidance. Invisible learning is what is absorbed by people through watching and listening to what is going on around them. Since sex is an important subject, young people are especially sensitive to the way adults behave sexually.

Furthermore, sex is a mystery, a puzzle that needs to be solved. Children have numerous unanswered questions. Many of these questions will, in the end, be answered by observing adults. It is worth remembering that young people learn from adults, not the other way around.

Friends

It is common knowledge that young people learn as much
about sex, if not more, from their friends as from anyone
else. On the whole, adults tend to be suspicious about this
learning. It is assumed that what children and teenagers
learn from their friends consists mainly of false or
misleading information. It is also assumed that it is
through friends and the peer group that myths about
sexuality circulate (such as 'you can't get pregnant if
you do it standing up').

Very little research evidence is available on this topic,
so, in fact, we don't really know much about what we
might call 'playground learning'. It seems probable that
there are both good and bad aspects of this. We certainly
need to recognise that friends have a very important part
to play in helping young people piece together the puzzle
of sex.

Let us look first at the positive aspects of playground
learning:

- Young people are less inhibited with their friends.
  This makes it possible for them to share anxieties
  and concerns, and to discuss difficult topics.
- Young people obtain support from each other. It is
  easier to talk about an embarrassing or awkward
  topic with someone, if you know they are facing the
  same problems.
- The peer group is a social arena. This means that some
  learning will take place through trying out different
  ways of behaving. Much learning about sex will
  occur, not by talking or listening, but by interacting
  with others, and discovering what works and what
  doesn't.

Of course, learning from friends is not always a good thing. It is certainly true that young people do not have all the facts.

They may lack information, or they may simply get things wrong. It is easy to see how one person's ignorance can get passed around a group of friends, magnifying the effect of a misunderstanding:

When I was in my primary school – I was about ten – we started sex education for the first time, which I thought was good, starting at that age. And you know, friends were talking about things on telly and that, and they were going round talking about periods and that in the playground. They were saying one can last for about six months, and all this lot. And you were getting really confused, and going home and telling your mum about this. I always remember being told that you get pregnant by a seed being put in a cup. That's how you got pregnant. So I got a bit confused over that, because I thought that for about two or three years. I wouldn't tell anyone that. I really felt embarrassed about that sort of thing. But that happens a lot. I know from my friends as well as they have told me that that happens.

16-year-old girl

Perhaps the most damaging feature of playground learning is social pressure. I have already given an example of young people believing that they ought to be sexually active, because it appears that so many of their friends are gaining sexual experience. Young people boast about and exaggerate the extent of their sexual activity, but the effect is to create pressure on many teenagers to hurry up and get on with it.

We need to understand more about the role of friends in the area of sexual learning. Friends can be an asset, a strength and a resource for young people. As adults, we need to identify more clearly the ways in which incorrect information gets passed around. This would then make it easier for teachers, parents and carers to counteract the effects, and to provide essential knowledge at key stages of development. Lastly, adults could help young people to resist social pressure by providing support, as well as by supplying the factual information that teenagers need to help them stand up to the peer group.

The media

Few subjects have caused more disagreement than the effects of the media on children and adolescents. Once again, this is a debate where, unfortunately, only the extreme positions receive much attention. Furthermore, most of the argument has revolved around the effects of violence, and little note has been taken of the effect of the media on the sexual attitudes and behaviour of the young.

It is clear that children and adolescents are receptive to, and are therefore likely to learn from, all aspects of the media. Here we must include not only TV and news-papers, but also magazines, films, books and videos. The big question is: What sort of learning takes place? Do young people absorb everything they watch and read? Are they prepared to believe whatever appears on television? This is what adults fear. However, there may be an alternative view. Perhaps young people are actually quite discriminating. Maybe they are only too well aware that television is television, not real life. It is possible that they are quite skilled at sorting out what is rubbish from what is useful. If this is the case, then perhaps the influence of the media is not so bad after all.

In fact, the truth probably lies somewhere in between these two positions. Age and maturity have something to do with it, for, obviously, the older the individual the more discriminating they are. In addition, it is probably true to say that people are more influenced by the media if they do not have alternative sources of information. Thus, for example, young people who have good sex education at school, as well as the chance to discuss sexual issues at home, will be better able to judge the accuracy of media information. Lastly, books, videos and magazines do not all carry the same weight. Information from a respected agony aunt in *Just Seventeen* is more likely to be believed than something one girl tells another in *Brookside*.

As with all sources of learning, there are advantages and disadvantages to the media. Some of the benefits are:

- Difficult topics can be addressed by responsible journalists and TV producers. In Britain, there have been examples of soaps dealing with topics which are not dealt with anywhere else.
- Agony aunts and uncles do provide information on topics which teachers and parents find difficult to tackle. Judging by the stream of letters and queries reaching these journalists, they are offering an important service to many thousands of young people.
- As with all things, learning gained from the media has to be placed in context. If media information is all that is available, this cannot be good. However, if it is one element of a wider picture, then the encouragement of imagination, the opportunity to learn about different worlds and different values, and the ability to compare

one's own experiences with those of other people all enhance the young person's learning.

In conclusion, we need to acknowledge that the media can have a powerful influence on young people. However, the extent of the influence depends on a number of factors. It is up to the parents and other adults to ensure:

- that different media are on offer. Sitting in front of the television day in and day out is not good for anyone. Books, films and magazines all provide alternative viewpoints.
- that the young person develops the ability to make judgements about what she or he is watching or reading. This skill can be developed by adults at home and at school.
- that the young person is not continually alone when exposed to the media. Any influence the media may have is undoubtedly diminished if the young person has the opportunity to discuss the material with others. Parents and other trusted adults are obviously of greatest importance in this respect.

Communication

This chapter is concerned with the way young people learn about sex. As we have seen, learning takes place in all sorts of ways, and stems from many different sources. In spite of this, it still remains true that the most powerful learning occurs as a result of communication between people. In the case of teenagers and sex, one critical aspect of communication is that which involves parents.

Research shows that, almost without exception, young people want more chances to talk with adults about sex and sexuality. When asked with which adults they would most like to discuss these matters, the great majority say their parents. If this is the case, why don't they? Because, as teenagers see it, their parents are too embarrassed or awkward to make such discussions possible.

Strangely, adults have a rather different perspective! The experience of most parents is that it is the young people who are the most embarrassed by the topic of sex. It is the teenagers who hold back, or find some excuse, or end up by saying 'don't bother mum, I know it all already'. So what can be done? First, a few things about communication.

Not all communication is verbal communication

You don't necessarily have to talk to someone to communicate with them. You can communicate your interest and concern to your children in many different ways. Leaving a good sex-education book or information leaflet around the house is one way of saying 'I want to help'. A squeeze on the shoulder when someone is upset, or simply an offer to go to the clinic or to the doctor together – these are types of communication that may be more effective than saying 'Okay, time to talk'.

Verbal communication is complicated, and involves a lot more than talking

Good communication is often described as a 'two-way street'. By this it is meant that if you want to communicate with someone, you have to listen as well as talk. Your teenager will be far more likely to concentrate on what you have to say if she or he knows that you are also prepared to listen. Listening and talking go hand in hand.

Closely linked with this is a third communication skill – making sure that you have been heard. After all, there's not much point in spending ten minutes reeling off a list of arguments to support your point of view, if the other person cannot hear what you have to say. In order to be heard, you have to choose the right time to express your opinion, you have to use an appropriate tone and language, and most important of all, you have to show that you are willing to listen to the other person too.

Understanding the skills of communication will help in overcoming some of the embarrassment of talking about sex. If you want to be able to communicate with your teenager about sex, or indeed about any difficult topic, here are some dos and don'ts.

Don't   expect to be able to sit down at the kitchen table and say 'Right, let's talk about the facts of life'. It won't work.

Do   be prepared to wait for the right time. This may be after a family event, a scene from TV, or when your daughter has had a row with her boyfriend.

Don't   try to cover all the issues at the same time. Take it slowly. Remember there *will* be other opportunities, as long as you don't force the pace.

Do   be prepared to share some of your own experiences. It is helpful for young people to learn that their parents didn't get it right the first time either.

Don't   go too far with this sort of disclosure. Your son or daughter wants to know you are human, not that you've had a super-human sex life!

Do   be prepared to make yourself available, even at inconvenient times. Teenagers are more likely to want to talk at midnight than at midday. This can be hard for parents, especially for those who have a long day ahead. Nonetheless, some 'heart to heart' talks are too important to be missed.

Don't   try to set the agenda yourself. Listen carefully to the clues that your teenager provides. She or he will find a way of telling you what's important at any particular time. You are more likely to be able to communicate about the subjects on the teenager's agenda, than about those on your own agenda. However, some give and take is possible, and you can always indicate that you have made space for the young person's concerns, so now it is time for them to do the same for you.

Do   be prepared to help with setting the boundaries of acceptable behaviour.

Teenagers may need you to help them sort out how far to go in their sexual behaviour. Be honest, and tell them what you think the limits are. This may come as a great relief to them.

Finally

Do   show your teenager some respect. Good communication is based on the belief that the other person is genuinely interested in who you are, and in what you have to say. If you can get that across to your daughter or son, there will be opportunities for genuine sharing between you.

Useful organisations

For information about sex education in schools, contact **The Sex Education Forum**, c/o National Children's Bureau, 8 Wakley Street, London EC1V 7QE. Tel: 020 7843 6052/6056. Email: sexedforum@ncb.org.uk

The fpa (formerly the Family Planning Association) provides a wide variety of services for parents and young people concerned with sexual health. It provides a confidential advice service and produces and distributes publications, videos and resources on sexual health and contraception. Address: 2–12 Pentonville Road, London N19FP. Helpline: 020 7837 4044.

Useful reading

Let's Talk about Sex by Robie H. Harris – Walker Books (1995). This book provides answers to the question pre-teens and teenagers ask about contraception, puberty, the body, families, contraception and sexual health.

Talking to Your Kids about Sex by Dr David Delvin and Christine Webber – fpa (2000). This amusing video for parents comes with a booklet offering tips and advice on how to tell your child about puberty, sex and relationships. Available from fpa direct, PO Box 1078, East Oxford DO, Oxfordshire OX4 6JE. Tel: 01865 719418.

The Parents' Pack – fpa (2000). This pack contains fpa booklets for young people as well as a parents' booklet, *Talking to Your Child about Sex*. Available from fpa direct (see above for details).

The Parentalk Guide to Your Child and Sex by Steve Chalke – Hodder and Stoughton (1999).

Useful websites

www.bbc.co.uk/worldservice/sexwise is a global on-line sex-education project including news reports and audio links to real people's experiences.

www.fpa.org.uk provides information about con-traception, sexual health, publications and resources for young people, parents and profes-sionals.

www.thesite.org looks at a range of issues that affect the lives of young people such as health, sex and relationships.

3

Sexual development in early adolescence

In this chapter, I will consider some aspects of sexual development which start to occur during or after puberty.

The topics I am going to cover include:

The need for privacy
Relationships with adults
Boys and girls are different
Masturbation
The fears and anxieties of adults
The fears and anxieties of teenagers

The need for privacy

One almost universal feature of adolescent behaviour, especially around the time of puberty, is the need for greater privacy. It is at this time that parents notice doors being locked, signs appearing which say 'no admittance', and longer queues for the bathroom. For some parents, this can seem like an unwelcome change. Suddenly, a girl or boy, once an open loving child with whom you could discuss anything at all, becomes a closed, private individual. You feel shut out, and this is an experience which can be very hurtful.

It is important to keep in mind that there are good reasons behind the need for privacy:

- **Sensitivity about bodily changes.** Young people may find the physical changes of puberty very unsettling. They may feel shy or awkward, or embarrassed about their bodies. As a result, they want to be sure that no one barges into the bathroom or bedroom while they are undressed.
- **Self-consciousness.** At this stage, teenagers be-come hypersensitive about their appearance. They may want to try out different hairstyles, or different clothes, and they may want to do this on their own. The mirror can become their best friend.
- **Sexuality.** The need for privacy may be related to the existence of new sexual feelings or fantasies. Your teenager may stick pictures of pop stars on his or her bedroom walls, or read teenage magazines secretly in bed. Young people need space and time alone to experience these early signs of sexual development.

While parents may find this need for privacy difficult to cope with, it is an essential part of growing up. Teenagers do need space and time on their own. They do need to be allowed privacy to explore their new internal world. Without this, they will feel pressured and harassed, and possibly bad-tempered!

It may seem to parents that the need for privacy is a sign that the child is lost to them, or doing something that has been forbidden. In fact, quite the opposite is true. Young people who are allowed some private space will be more likely to seek out their parents when they need them. Teenagers who feel that their parents are always intruding are the ones who move away as soon as they can:

> *She often says to me: 'Why don't you talk about your problems?' I say 'I do, I just don't talk to you. I talk to my friends'. I have talked to my mum about things, but not at the time they're happening. I tell her about them after they've happened, after I sorted it out for myself what's happening. I still think she wants me to tell her, but I can't.*
>
> 15-year-old girl

Relationships with adults

Adults, and especially parents and carers, have a major role to play in the life of the teenager. A supportive and concerned adult can make all the difference when the young person is unhappy or upset. A sensitive teacher can provide a lifeline when things seem very bleak. An aunt, uncle or other relative can offer advice or information which enables the young person to solve a pressing personal problem. These are just a few examples of the ways in which adults can be influential at key moments.

More generally, though, adults matter to adolescents for a number of reasons:

- However much bravado there is, young people are still dependent on adults for many of their emotional needs.
- Teenagers respond best when there are boundaries and limits. They need to know how far they can go. Only adults can provide this structure.
- Young people need role models. As they face questions about their identity, teenagers need models and examples upon which to base their choices.
- Adolescents need a reference point. Research shows that, as far as self-image is concerned, young people are more influenced by how their parents judge them than by any other factor.
- Teenagers need encouragement and support. Apart from intelligence, the factor which has most influence on school achievement is parental interest and involvement with homework.

Some parents may find the proposition that 'adults do matter' rather difficult to believe. Faced with a moody and resentful 14-year-old, it may seem that the very opposite is true. Nonetheless, you are important. You do make a difference. Your teenager needs you just as much as she or he did in early childhood. It is only that the needs are expressed in different ways – often heavily disguised!

Not surprisingly, adults find moodiness and hostility difficult to deal with. Sometimes, parents say that their child's behaviour simply doesn't make sense. Teenagers seem to be a sort of Jekyll and Hyde – sunny and smiling one moment, impossible the next. It is worth remembering that behaviour of this sort is very common among young people, especially in the early years of adolescence.

Here are some of the reasons:

- **Hormones.** During puberty a major change takes place in your adolescent's hormonal balance. Adjusting to these alterations is not easy. Some moodiness is probably a direct result of hormonal variation.
- **Transition.** Your adolescent faces a difficult task – moving from childhood to adulthood over a long-drawn-out period. During much of this time, they won't quite know where they stand. Mature or immature? Grown up or child-like? Much of the puzz-ling behaviour reflects this uncertainty.
- **Breaking away.** Another challenge faced by your teenager is that they need to create more of an emotional distance from you. This is a natural part of growing up. Nonetheless, breaking away is never easy, and sometimes young people seem to over-react. They may give the impression of wanting to reject you altogether. Keep in mind that this is only a stage. It is no more than a strategy to help them with the task of growing up.

We need to understand a little bit about adolescent development, and the important role that adults play at this stage, if we are to make sense of adolescent sexuality. Sexuality is an especially sensitive topic. It is a central feature of development at this time. Yet, it is a subject fraught with embarrassment and anxiety. Young people need information, advice, support and the opportunity to discuss many of the issues associated with sexuality, and, yet, it may be impossible for them to do so with their parents.

Many of the points outlined in the previous section are relevant here. Adults are very important indeed where sexuality is concerned, and yet teenage behaviour may seem to suggest the opposite. It is up to parents and carers to overcome the barriers, and recognise the role they can play. It *is* possible to provide information and advice, it *is* possible to be supportive and it *is* possible to have an influence. Parents and carers *can* be active and involved, and we will be looking at how this can be done in subsequent chapters of this book.

Boys and girls are different

This may seem to be stating the obvious, but it is necessary to underline the fact that early sexual development is experienced quite differently by males and females. Many parents reading this will have both daughters and sons. Yet, surprisingly, and all too frequently, families fail to appreciate that the needs of girls and boys are not going to be the same. The difference of gender has important implications, and requires different approaches. Sensitivity on the part of parents and carers to the characteristics of female and male development at this age is crucial. Let me outline some of these characteristics:

- The physical changes associated with puberty may have more of an impact on girls than on boys. Certainly, boys do not have to adjust to any experience equivalent to menstruation.
- Girls express greater dissatisfaction with their bodies than boys do during early adolescence. Feelings of dissatisfaction for girls centre particularly on breast size, weight and facial characteristics.
- Girls feel that they are the target of more media pressure than boys, in relation to what constitutes ideal weight, height and shape. There is more stereotyping of female beauty, and girls are under more pressure

than boys to diet and to conform to what is considered
to be 'the perfect woman'.

- Girls' and boys' friendships are different. Boys'
  friendships are centred on shared activities, while
  girls are more likely to have close relationships in
  which feelings can be discussed.
- Girls get more support from their friends in this way.
  This is especially important, since boys have less opportunity to express emotion. They may therefore be
  more vulnerable when things go wrong.
- Boys are more likely to be affected by a lack of appropriate role models. The fact that so much parenting is
  done by women does put boys at a disadvantage.
  Where there is an absence of a close relationship
  with an adult male, the boy's developing sexuality
  may suffer.
- Parents are more likely to be worried about the personal
  safety of girls than of boys. This can result in girls experiencing greater restrictions on their freedom, which
  may be a cause of conflict in some families.
- Finally, the distribution of power in sexual relationships is still unequal. This means that in many
  situations it remains difficult for girls to take control
  of events. This has particular relevance to the use of
  contraceptives, and to decisions and choices about
  how far to go in sexual activity.

These issues will not necessarily apply in all circumstances. Nonetheless, if parents and carers can keep in
mind the differing needs of girls and boys, they will
undoubtedly be more likely to be able to offer the right
type of support for the teenagers in their family:

*I think up until puberty for girls there's this
wonderful feeling that you can climb anywhere, run*

anywhere, do anything you like, and then you're brought up short by this equipment that starts changing and slows you down and makes you weepy and bleeds on you and it goes out of your control ... A lot of girls around 11, they actually can run faster than boys, and they're more verbal and they're cheeky and they feel they can do anything. And suddenly, you know, the shutters come down about what's possible on certain days of the month. I think that's something that has to be talked about to girls in order for them to place it and allow it to happen to them without allowing it to stop them doing things they still want to do.

Mother of two daughters

Masturbation

Masturbation is a topic that is rarely discussed. It is unlikely to feature in any sex-education lesson, and it is hardly ever mentioned in the home. Indeed, it is even one of the few subjects that is avoided when young people are with their friends. Why should this be so?

It has to be concluded that strong taboos still operate where masturbation is concerned. How many couples, I wonder, have discussed the subject with each other? It is not quite clear why masturbation is such a difficult topic. Is it simply a hangover from the Victorian era? Is it because attaining sexual gratification on your own is still in some way seen as shameful? Masturbation is certainly a good example of the fact that, although there have been huge changes in sexual attitudes and behaviour since the 1960s, there are still some areas where major inhibitions remain.

Masturbation is a perfectly normal and healthy expression of sexual need. It is a pleasurable activity which has no harmful or negative consequences. Surveys of sexual behaviour show that there is wide variation between individuals in the frequency of masturbation. Some masturbate often, some rarely, some not at all. Approximately two-thirds of women have masturbated at some time or another while almost all men have done so. Many people masturbate at the same time as having a satisfying sex life with a partner.

There are still many myths about masturbation, and teenagers are more likely than adults to worry about some of these. No one any longer believes Victorian notions such as that masturbation leads to blindness. Nonetheless, many people still do have anxieties about it. Boys may fear that masturbation will affect their virility or their capacity to produce semen. Girls may worry their clitoris or vagina will become less responsive to stimulation when they have sex with another person. Both boys and girls may feel ashamed that they have become aroused on their own, rather than with a partner.

Young people need reassurance about masturbation. They need to know that it is healthy and harmless. They also need to know that it is something that most people do at some stage in their lives. Masturbation is a normal outlet for sexual arousal. If adults have the opportunity, they should make sure that teenagers know the facts about this subject.

The fears and anxieties of parents

I want to conclude this chapter by outlining some of the more common fears experienced by both adults and teenagers in relation to adolescent sexuality. All of us have worries and anxieties, and one useful way to deal with these is to be open and honest about them. Let us look first at the parents' perspective.

Talking about sex encourages teenagers to go and try it

Many adults worry that sex education, or discussions in the home, act as a green light for young people to go out and experiment. This is an understandable concern, but the facts indicate that the opposite is true. The most conclusive evidence comes from comparisons of teenage pregnancy rates in different countries. Where teenage pregnancy rates are lowest there is extensive sex education, and freely available contraceptive services for young people – as in Holland and Sweden.

Furthermore, research in Britain and in the United States indicates that young people are more likely to delay their first sexual experience if they come from a home where sex is discussed openly. If you still have doubts, remember this. Sex is a topic of public debate. Your teenager is going to be talking about it anyway. Isn't it better that he or she talks about it with you?

Sex is too embarrassing to discuss

Many people are too embarrassed to discuss sex, especially with their own children. However, there are many ways of communicating, and not all of them involve sitting down and talking. Suggestions for different approaches to communication have already been outlined in the previous chapter. There is also more about this in Chapter 9 at the end of the book.

Your teenager may know more than you

This is a possibility, especially in relation to topics such as HIV/AIDS or drugs. Be honest with your daughter or son, and be prepared to accept that you are not the fountain of all wisdom! If you make it clear that you are keen to learn, they will be happy to share their knowledge with you. They will also then be more likely to take on board what you have to teach them. There may also be situations where you are both ignorant. Perhaps neither of you knows much about sexually transmitted infections (STIs). Offer to get a book or leaflet out of the library, so that you can learn together. You may be surprised how interested the young person is in this approach.

Your son or daughter will get involved in a sexual relationship before he or she is ready

There is little a parent or carer can do to stop a young person becoming sexually active, if that is what they are determined to do. However, there is an enormous amount an adult can do to make sure that the teenager is well informed, and properly prepared. This applies both to physical and emotional preparation for sex. Parents can also ensure that girls and boys have access to an appropriate contraceptive. In summary, you can't stop them doing it, but you can help them to be safe.

Your son or daughter will be subjected to peer pressure from unsuitable friends

Peer pressure is a powerful force which operates among all of us, but it may be that teenagers are more susceptible to this pressure, especially in the years following puberty. It is important for you to know that some young people are better at resisting peer pressure than others, and it is quite clear that adults play a key role here. Support from parents is one of the things which is most helpful to young people in resisting this pressure. Try not to criticise your children's friends, or exclude them from your home. The more they are part of your life, the more influence you will have and the more likely you are to be able to keep an eye on what's going on.

The fears and anxieties of teenagers

Finally, let us look at some of the fears of young people themselves. If you as a parent or carer can be aware of these, there may be ways in which you can help.

'My body is not normal'

This is probably the most common fear of all. In fact, there are few teenagers who have not worried at some time or other about their bodies, and how they compare with their friends. Two things are worth bearing in mind here:

● First, everyone is different. There is no such thing as normal where bodies are concerned. People develop at different rates, and in different ways. No two girls have exactly the same breasts. No two boys have exactly the same penises. Your son or daughter does not need to worry about being different.

- Second, the way we develop around puberty bears very little relation to how we are as mature adults. Whether your teenager is slow or fast in her or his development will be forgotten within a few years. It may seem very important to the girl or boy to be in step with the rest of the class. This is understandable. In the long run, however, the difference between friends at 12 or 13 will have been com-pletely forgotten when they are 16 or 18.

'I think about sex too much'

Many young people find that, as they move into adolescence, the subject of sex begins to dominate their thinking. As with everything to do with sex, there are great differences between individuals. Some young people may spend a lot of their time having daydreams or fantasies about sex. They may lie in bed thinking sexual thoughts, they may masturbate or they may seek out books or videos having sexual themes. On the other hand, there are others of the same age who do none of these things.

There is no such thing as thinking about sex too much. We all have different levels of sexual need, and different levels of arousal. Each of us has to come to terms with the way we are, and find healthy and satisfactory outlets for our sexual desires.

'Should I have done "it" by now?'

In our society, there is considerable pressure on young people to become sexually active. This pressure comes from the media, from the adult world and it also comes from the peer group.

There is also much exaggeration, by both girls and boys, about the extent of their sexual experience. Nonetheless, many feel that they need to have done certain things in order 'to keep in with the crowd'. This can create powerful pressures, and make life very uncomfortable for some teenagers.

Two things can help young people to resist peer pressure:

- Having access to good sensible information about sex. For example, it helps teenagers to know that no more than one in five 15-year-old girls have had sexual intercourse in Britain today. This is an aver-age figure, so there is going to be a lot of variation depending on the part of the country we are talking about. However, the key thing to emphasise is that, while young people may think that 'everyone is doing it', the reality is very different.
- As I have already said, support from parents is crucial to help the young person resist peer pressure. If teenagers know that their parents respect and value them, then they are likely to have the strength to stand up for what they believe in. It is also a bonus for them to know that help from adults will be available if it is needed.

'Am I too easily aroused?'/'Am I too frigid?'

It is not surprising that teenagers worry about their ability to become sexually aroused. After all, sexual experiences will be quite new to them, and young people are bound to be uncertain about how their bodies function, and whether what is going to happen to them is the same as what is happening to everyone else.

Many boys find getting an erection extremely embarrassing, especially if it occurs in public. Boys may be surprised at how easily they become excited, and alarmed that this can happen on a bus, in a school lesson or in the supermarket. Sexual arousal for girls is much less visible, and so there may be different fears. Even so, early experiences of erect nipples or of becoming wet around the vaginal area may be worrying too. Girls may feel convinced that such things are visible, even if they are not.

Anxieties about frigidity or impotence are also commonplace, being directly linked to questions of sexual performance. Boys may worry that they won't be able to do 'it', and will thus become a laughing stock. Girls may worry that unless they are sexually responsive they will be unable to attract or hold on to a boyfriend. In most cases, fears of this sort recede as young people become sexually experienced. If the fears persist, then some help or advice may be necessary. Suitable organisations are listed at the end of the chapters of this book:

I remember I was quite worried before. You know, when you sort of lose your virginity you think 'I've got to put on a big, a good show'. And then when you do actually get round to it, you usually blow it very quickly and you think 'Is this it? Is this what it's all about?' Worrying that the girl has probably done it before, and thinks you're an absolute failure, and she's gonna tell everyone, and that all goes through your head. It's all that macho kind of thing, that you've got to be able to perform, you've got to be you know big and hard and tough and all this kind of rubbish.

19-year-old man

'Am I gay, lesbian or straight?'

It is a tragedy that in our society we are still unable to talk openly about issues to do with sexual orientation. We ought to be able to offer young people information and advice about heterosexuality and homosexuality, as well as the opportunity to discuss any concerns they have. Sadly, we cannot do so, and thus questions about sexual orientation go unanswered.

Although we cannot be sure, it is probable that many heterosexual teenagers worry at some stage if they are gay or lesbian. Similarly those who are homosexual worry about how their parents and friends will react, how much they can say to the adults around them and so on. We do urgently need a more responsible and sensitive approach to this issue. I will say more about the subject in Chapter 7.

Useful reading

Adolescence – The survival Guide for Parents and Teenagers by Dr Tony Smith and Elizabeth Fenwick – Dorling Kindersley (1998). Includes case studies and true to life dialogues to help improve communication and answer questions.

Teenagers and Sexuality. This tape pack is produced by the Trust for the Study of Adolescence (TSA). It includes topics such as physical changes, first relationships and sexual identity. Available from TSA Publishing Ltd, 23 New Road, Brighton, BN1 1WZ. Tel: 01273 693311.

Useful websites

www.tsa.uk.com provides information about the work of the Trust for the Study of Adolescence and has details of a wide range of publications for parents and teenagers.

4

First relationships

In this chapter, I will explore the issues associated with early sexual relationships. Clearly, the first time an individual experiences sex represents a major landmark. It is something we remember vividly, and for most it symbolises an important step towards adulthood. The idea of 'losing one's virginity' can be a scary event, an obstacle to be overcome, a challenge, a longed-for moment. Boys and girls may feel differently about it, but one thing is certain; for most in our society, it is the closest we come to a 'rite of passage', a ritual that marks the fact that we have, at last, reached maturity. Early sexual experience is also likely to involve a range of new feelings. Understanding and support from parents at this time can be crucial.

In this chapter, I will cover:

Love and romance

Readiness for sex

Contraception

Personal safety

Essential messages for parents to emphasise

Love and romance

There are many different ways in which a first sexual
relationship can happen. In many cases – even today –
young people do not start having sex until they feel
something special for their partner. While the impression
is given by the media that teenagers are spending most of
their time hopping in and out of bed with anyone they
fancy, the facts are rather different. The majority of
young people:

● have sex within a lasting relationship;
● have sex with only one person at a time;
● believe that sex should only be part of an important
  relationship.

Most recent figures in Britain show that up to the age of 16
only 20% of girls (one in five) have had sexual intercourse,
while approximately 25% of boys at this age claim that
they are sexually experienced. These figures are higher
than they were 20 years ago, and there has certainly
been a lowering of the age of first sexual activity. Young
people today are having sex at an earlier age than they
were in the 1970s and 1980s.

In spite of this, however, the figures are still lower
than many parents imagine. Put another way, the figures
show that by the age of 16 four out of five girls (80%) have

not had a first sexual experience. Thus the great majority
of girls in Britain today are still virgins when they reach
the age of 16. This is not the sort of headline seen in the
tabloid newspapers! It should also be noted that there are
marked regional variations. While in some inner-city
areas the figures may be higher than this, in other parts
of the country fewer than one in eight 16-year-old girls
will be sexually active. These facts are important, and help
us to get some perspective on an issue about which many
people have strong feelings.

Unfortunately there is little good research which tells
us about patterns of sexual activity among younger
teenagers. Clearly, there are many different ways in
which members of this age group start to become sexually
active. Some will have a first sexual experience at a party
or other social event. This may be associated with alcohol
or drug use. It may be a 'one-night stand', and have little
meaning in terms of a long-term relationship. However,
the first sexual experience for many young people happens
only after a lengthy sequence of other events. Two
teenagers may go out together, or spend time together at
the weekends. They begin to share hopes and ideas with
each other and, if things progress, they begin to develop a
feeling that this is a special relationship. At the same time,
they begin to be affectionate with each other. They will
hold hands, kiss and want to be physically close to each
other. This may lead to further sexual exploration, which
may be accompanied by a sense of 'being in love':

*I've got a friend who's 13 at the moment who's quite a
good friend. She always tends to act much older, but
she's 13 and she always sort of goes out with a boy and
sort of a week later she'll go 'I'm in love' and she'll be
serious and I sort of laugh at her really. I know that a
week later she'll have given up on him and go out with*

another boy. Lots of times at this age I think, like, feelings can come out a lot more and it can make you feel like there's something going there, like love or some-thing, even after only a week of going out with somebody. So it takes quite a long time to settle down and sort of realise that not every little feeling is love. It might be just lust, or you know, friendship, or some-thing like that in a different way. It takes quite a time to get that sorted out.

15-year-old girl

Of course, young people may believe they are in love with someone without their being any physical contact. Alternatively, they may have sex together without any special feeling between them. As we have said, first sex-ual experiences can occur in many different ways, and in a moment we will consider how parents should respond, and what role they have to play. First, though, I will consider readiness for sex.

Readiness for sex

Young people today grow up in a world where attitudes to sex are very confusing indeed. As I have indicated in Chapter 2, from their very early years, children are trying to make sense of the puzzle of sex, and want to know what it is all about.

A hundred years ago there was much less public discussion about sex. Sex outside marriage was frowned upon, divorce was hard to obtain and contraceptives were not available in the way they are today. There was less questioning of the meaning of sex, since it had its place within the framework of marriage and childbearing. Today, however, those certainties do not exist, and no one is quite sure how to explain the meaning of sex. Is it no more than a pleasurable activity, rather like having a good meal? Does it matter if it has nothing to do with love, or trust, or commitment to another person? Can sex be as good with a stranger as with a long-term partner? These are the sorts of questions that young people would like to ask. Unfortunately, they are rarely answered, or indeed discussed, by parents or other adults.

As I have indicated, it is to adult behaviour that young people look for solutions to the puzzle. What do they see? They see many families disrupted by divorce or separation, often because one partner falls in love with someone else. They see neighbours, relatives, public figures having affairs. They see adults openly disagreeing about things like sex education, the provision of contraceptives for teenagers and so on.

The effect of all this must be:

- to create uncertainty;
- to underline the fact that many adults will sacrifice an enormous amount for sexual gratification;
- to lead young people to question whether adults have any authority to give them advice;
- to conclude that they need to make their own decisions about the meaning of sex.

I raise these issues because one of the questions most frequently asked by young people is: 'When is someone ready to have sex?' It is one of the most difficult to answer, but, also, it is one that cannot be answered without having some view on the meaning of sex.

After all, if you think sex is simply about bodily

pleasure, then young people might as well have sex for fun, whenever they feel like it. Of course, in our society very few of us take that view. Most of us believe that sex should be delayed at least until the individual is emotionally mature enough to take precautions and cope with the consequences of a sexual relationship. Indeed, most parents would probably say that they hope their son or daughter would wait for as long as possible. Some may believe that sex should only take place once two people are engaged, or at least intending to get married. Today, this is a minority view, but it is not uncommon:

> *Well, I'm Christian, so technically I should say you should not have sex until after marriage, but I also don't believe in hard and fast social rules, so I think the most sensible thing to say is when you feel ready and comfortable. For me, I think that would be when I'd left home. While I'm still at home, I still feel too much, even though sort of technically old enough and all the rest of it, I still feel too much part of a family and a child within that family. So I think it's important to get it right. I mean when you feel ready, and when you think you are old enough.*
>
> 16-year-old girl

For complicated reasons, the sexual activity of our children is something that most adults find difficult to deal with. It helps to be aware of some of our complex feelings, especially our reluctance to accept the sexuality of our daughters and sons. As adults, we need to acknowledge our own strong feelings if the advice we give to young people is to be of any use at all.

So what do you say when asked 'Mum, how old do I have to be before I can have sex?' To some extent the answer will depend on the values of the parents. Some may say 'Not until you've left home' or 'Not until you're engaged to be married'. The danger here, of course, is that any message that sounds like 'I don't want you to do it' may act as a challenge or provocation. When they ask this question, young people do not want to be told that sex is forbidden to them. If this is what they hear, it may just be the signal they need to go off and try it.

What teenagers do want is an open and honest discussion about early sexual activity. This should be combined with a recognition that at 16, or 15, or even 14, they are old enough to have sex, and there is not much that can stop them if they are really determined.

This may sound depressing to parents who worry about their teenager's health, safety and welfare. However, there are many ways in which parents can be helpful. There is much that parents can do to emphasise the risks of early sexual activity, and there are strong reasons why young people should delay. Outlining these in a non-judgemental way can make a real difference to a young person.

These are some of the things you can say:

- You should not have sex until you feel sure that you can trust the other person.
- You should not have sex until *you* feel ready. If the other person is putting pressure on you – then say no.
- You should not have sex until you can discuss and decide about contraception together.
- You should not have sex until you can handle the emotional feelings that you may experience.
- You should not have sex until you are absolutely sure that you and your partner will be protected against pregnancy and sexually transmitted infections (STIs).

These answers do not cover all the things that might come up in a conversation with your teenager. They will not provide a foolproof guide for a young person who wants answers on this issue. However, these responses will be helpful. They will enable a parent or carer to concentrate on the most obvious criteria that could be used to make a decision about readiness for sex. At the very least, they will show that sex and relationships are linked together. If expressed in the right way, these points will encourage your daughter or son to stop and think.

Contraception

It is sometimes very difficult for parents to be clear about their role in relation to contraception. How far can parents go in trying to make sure that a teenager is going to use the right contraceptive? Should a father buy condoms for his son? Should a mother take her daughter to the GP, or to the family-planning clinic?

> *I remember when I wanted to go on the pill, it took me weeks and weeks to ask my mum. I remember I was like waiting for the right moment for weeks like, and she eventually just said 'yeah, all right then, I'll take you down to the clinic then'. And I was going aaaaagh! I had to wait until we went on holiday and wait till my mum was a bit drunk and after we'd had a meal to eventually ask her, but she was fine about it. It's so embarrassing.*
>
> 18-year-old young woman

The fact is that parents and carers are caught in a trap here. If they try and help with contraception, they may believe they are encouraging sexual activity, or they may fear that they will be accused of interfering in something that is private. On the other hand, if they don't do anything, they experience all the anxiety of not being sure that the teenager is taking the proper precautions.

It is my view, and the view of all professionals in this field, that parents do have a role here, a very important role indeed. The reasons that parents give themselves for not doing anything are often excuses, as we can see if we look at them more closely.

To give advice about contraception will encourage sexual behaviour

There is absolutely no evidence that this is true. To think like this assumes that there are no other influences on young people. Your teenager will be worrying about these questions, and looking around for advice, whether you give it or not. Isn't it better that the advice comes from you, rather than from someone else?

To give advice about contraception is to intrude upon something that is private

Whether this is the case or not depends entirely on how the subject is approached. If the parent tries to take over, treating the teenager like an irresponsible child, it will not go down too well! If the parent treads cautiously, offering advice and support when and if the young person wants it, then this is likely to be more acceptable.

The question of contraception is a difficult one for young people. They do need assistance to get it right. While some find their way to user-friendly clinics, where they can have a full and frank discussion with a

family-planning nurse, these young people are probably
in the minority. More often, teenagers do not find it easy
to get good advice, and it is here that parents can play such
a key role. Questions that young people are likely to ask
will include some of the following:

'Which contraceptive should I use?'

Many girls worry about whether using the pill will have
side effects, or a long-term impact on their health. Others
may have heard that there are different types of contraceptive pill, but not know about the differences between
them. For boys, there may be concerns about the type of
condom to choose. What is the advantage of one sort over
another? Are they all lubricated? Are there different sizes,
and how do you choose which size is right? Should you use
ones that have a smell, or a taste? Such questions may
seem trivial, but they can seem like matters of life and
death to an anxious 16-year-old.

Parents and carers should make sure that young
people have the information they need to make sensible
decisions. This includes knowledge about newer contraceptive methods, such as the morning-after pill (also
known as emergency contraception), and the female
condom. While I do not discuss here the details of
different types of contraceptive, it is worth noting that
emergency contraception is now widely available. It may
also be particularly useful for teenagers, especially if they
have sex in an unplanned manner, as for example at a
party. Emergency contraception can be purchased by
anyone aged 16 or over at most chemists. It is also
available from some school nurses, and from any family-
planning clinic, young person's clinic or Brook clinic.
Emergency contraception must be taken within three
days, and is most effective if it is taken within 24 hours

of the woman having had sex. Further details may be obtained from the FPA, from Brook, or from other sources listed at the back of this chapter.

'How can I get hold of contraceptives?'

I have already mentioned the availability of emergency contraception. Condoms are also widely available, and in some places are provided free for young people. However, getting the pill or a diaphragm may pose more of a problem for a teenager, especially someone under the age of 16. Anxiety or embarrassment about making an appointment, or being recognised by someone at the clinic, can prevent young people from taking that crucial step.

Parents or carers can provide really important support here by giving gentle encouragement, by giving advice about where to go or by offering to accompany a young person to the clinic or doctor.

At the very least, adults should be aware of the location of the nearest young people's sexual-health service, and should make sure that their teenager knows this address.

'Even if I have a contraceptive, how can I make sure we use it?'

This is one of the biggest worries for young people. The negotiation between partners over the use of contraceptives requires self-confidence, maturity and good communication. These characteristics are unlikely to exist for teenagers in the early stages of sexual exploration. To be able to talk about such things with a trusted adult could be of enormous help.

It is difficult for young people to plan their sexual behaviour, and to be prepared. It is difficult enough for adults, so it should be no surprise to us to recognise the obstacles faced by teenagers. It may help parents and carers to look briefly at some of these obstacles:

- Young people may feel that using a contraceptive will spoil the magic moment. The common fear is that stopping to put on a condom or fiddling around with a diaphragm and some jelly will interfere with sex.
- Young people may feel ashamed of planning for sex. They may feel embarrassed or awkward about this, believing that to be seen to have planned for sex will put them in a bad light. This is a particular problem for girls.
- Young people may not know how to get access to contraceptives. This is a point which has already been mentioned. More information about access should be available in schools, youth clubs and other settings. Parents can make sure that information about where to go is in a prominent location at home.
- Young people may have sex infrequently, or it may happen quite unexpectedly. Obviously, planning in such circumstances is unlikely. It is precisely because of this possibility that is is worth talking to your teenager about contraception, even if they are not involved in a steady relationship.

Personal safety

This may be a good place to introduce the topic of personal safety. This represents one of the biggest fears

that parents have, particularly at the time that their teenagers are first becoming sexually active. Parents and
carers will have different feelings about boys and girls,
and will almost certainly feel more protective and more
concerned about the safety of girls than of boys. This is
not always easy to deal with. While some daughters may
accept, and even welcome, their parents' concern, others
are resentful, if they feel they have to live a more
restricted life than their brothers or male cousins.
Parents may worry that girls are more vulnerable. However, boys too can be victims of violence, and it is important in thinking about personal safety to remember
that everyone, male and female, needs to be sensible
and to avoid undue risk.

Parents and carers need to tread a fine line here. Being
too overprotective can cause young people to ignore good
advice. On the other hand, making the assumption that
young people will automatically know what to do and how
to avoid danger is not helpful either. As with all things,
parents will have most influence if they tread carefully,
and treat the young person as a 'trainee adult' rather
than as a child who needs instruction. Show some trust
in the young person, and in their good sense, but at the
same time ensure that they know some basic rules about
personal safety.

Let us look at some of the issues involved in personal
safety. First, the effects of drugs and alcohol. This is, of
course, a subject in itself, and suggestions for further
reading may be found at the end of the chapter. In the
present context, it needs to be clearly recognised, by both
adults and teenagers, that using drugs and/or alcohol
creates additional risk if sexual activity is taking place. It
is a sad fact that a high proportion of unplanned teenage
pregnancies occur as a result of the girl either having had
too much to drink or having used drugs. Using drugs or
alcohol impairs judgement. Using these substances makes

it that much more difficult for the teenager and his/her sexual partner to be sure they are properly protected.

There is only one conclusion. Sex should only take place with someone the teenager trusts, in a setting where the two individuals can be sure that they are both safe.

Being out alone at night is another way in which the teenager can be exposed to risk. There are a variety of ways in which parents can help. Don't leave things to chance. Do make sure that your teenager has a way to get home from a party or late-night event. Do make it clear that if something goes wrong, you will find a way of providing help. Do help your teenager plan journeys if she or he is travelling alone and at night.

Finally, if your teenager has to pass through places which may be unsafe – certain areas of big cities, for example, or along a lonely country lane – then offer to pay for a taxi, or arrange some other form of reliable transport. To some, this may seem like unnecessary nannying. Nonetheless, parents and carers can play a role where personal safety is concerned. Do make sure you have a thorough discussion on the subject:

There's nothing you can do to prevent a physical attack on an innocent young female by some slob of 16 stone. That is why I fear the rape situation. The only preventative measures, if that is possible, is to avoid being in areas where it's most likely to happen – walking alone at night. We've seen on television and the press this last year what hap-pens in railway compartments. Basically you try to encourage your adolescent daughter to be in places where there are people. People tend to form a safety network – a safety net that isn't there when you are on your own.
                                    Father of two daughters

In thinking about personal safety, we need also to address the issue of rape and assault. A terrible thing like this might happen out of the blue. It may occur simply because someone happens to be in a particular place at a particular time. Nonetheless, there are a variety of things that young women, and young men as well, can do to make themselves less vulnerable. We have already mentioned two of these: to be careful with drink and drugs, and to think ahead if anyone is going to be out alone at night. We can add others to this list, some of which apply particularly to young women, but it is important not to see this issue as one solely for females:

- it is useful to carry a personal alarm;
- a class in self-protection can be a good idea;
- young women should not go out with an older man on her own on a blind date;
- young women should treat all blind dates with great caution;
- young people should avoid travelling alone in the carriage of a train or tube;
- young women should not travel in a car on their own with an unknown man or group of men – this applies especially after a party, or other late-night event;
- young women should be extremely cautious about the messages they send, if they are out with some-one they do not know.

It is important for both girls and boys to know that there are things people can do in relation to personal safety. Nothing anyone can do will keep them perfectly safe. However, all of us can reduce the level of danger to which we are exposed. Sharing this with your daughter or son will prove a valuable exercise.

Essential messages for parents to emphasise

I want to conclude this chapter by looking at some of the key messages that parents and carers may want to convey in discussions with their teenagers. I have selected a number of points which, in my experience, seem to recur time and time again. Parents cannot hope to be influential in all areas of teenage behaviour. Nor can they expect their children to pay attention to everything that adults consider important. It is for this reason that it is worthwhile concentrating on a few central issues, particularly those which are relevant to the concerns, questions and anxieties that commonly trouble teenagers.

Sex does not make or break a good relationship

Many young people fear that, unless they are willing to have sex with someone they care about, the relationship will soon end. It is important to talk this through with your teenager. If the relationship between a girl and boy is a good one, then whether they have sex or not is something that can be worked out gradually. If a boy says to a girl that he will only stay with her is she has sex with him, then he is not worth hanging on to.

If you are not sure, say no

This is a point that cannot be emphasised enough. No one should be pressurised into sex. A teenager needs sufficient support from adults so that he or she feels confident enough to resist unwelcome advances.

Contraception is a joint responsibility

Young people, of both genders, should have this message up in large letters on their bedroom wall! The only way a relationship can be genuinely equal is for there to be shared responsibility for contraception, as well as for all other sexual decisions.

Boys should be encouraged to see that they have a role to play in ensuring their personal safety and that of their partners

Boys need to acknowledge that personal safety is not only a matter for females. In addition to taking care of themselves, they can also contribute to the personal safety of girls by making sure that they get home safely after a date, by not taking advantage if a girl has had something to drink, and by accepting that where sex is concerned 'no' means 'no'.

Pregnancy and sexually transmitted infections are a possibility

When you are young it is only too easy to believe that it won't happen to you. The responsibility of adults is to get across to young people that it can happen to anyone. Sex during adolescence can involve risk. No one should be allowed to forget that.

Parents are not obsessed with teenage sex

Young people often feel that their parents are preoccupied with the subject. One girl said in an interview 'My parents don't seem to talk about anything else. They are always asking me "Am I doing it yet?" They may be obsessed with sex, but I'm not.' The problem here is that parents allow their anxieties to show through. These anxieties mean that you may think about the sexuality of your son or daughter a lot, and this comes over as an obsession.

There is also a question of trust involved. Teenagers who sense that their parents are consistently asking questions about their sex life are made to feel that they are not trusted. If at all possible, you want to create exactly the opposite impression. The more your teenager feels trusted, the more likely she or he is to to share concerns with you.

You will be there, no matter what

Of all the messages that parents need to get across, this one is more important than any other. If teenagers know that whatever happens their parents will be there to support them, then much trouble and strife will be avoided. What do parents want? They want to be loved and respected, they want good communication and they want a continuing influence over their son or daughter. These things are most likely to occur if young people believe:

- that they are valued by their parents;
- that they will not be judged too harshly, even if they make mistakes;
- that they will be supported, even if they get into trouble.

Useful organisations

Brook provides free, confidential sex advice and contraception to all young people. It also provides advice to parents. For your nearest centre contact Brook at Studio 421, Highgate Studios 51–79 Highgate Road, London NW5 1TL. Tel: 0800 0185 023
Email: information@brookcentres. org.uk

Sexwise is a free helpline for young people aged 12-18 which offers advice and guidance on all sorts of sexuality and sexual health issues, including contraception, abortion, relationships and pregnancy. Tel: 0800 28 29 30.

Useful reading

Is Everybody Doing it? – fpa (2000). A full colour, highly illustrated booklet dealing with issues involved in starting a sexual relationship and using contraception. Available from fpa direct, PO Box 1078, East Oxford DO, Oxfordshire OX4 6JE. Tel: 01865 719418.

Living with a Teenager by Suzie Hayman – Piatkus (1998). Packed with insights and strategies to help understand your teenager's needs. How to negotiate, compromise and foster confidence.

Teenagers in the Family: Skills for Parents by John Coleman (2001). This video is based on real-life experiences faced by teenagers and their families, and contains advice and support for parents. Available from the Trust for the Study of Adolescence, 23 New Road, Brighton, BN1 1WZ. Tel: 01273 693311.

Bliss, The Smart Girl's Guide to Sex by Kerry Parnell; *The Smart Girl's Guide to Boys* by Maria Coole – Piccadilly Press (2000). Provide facts and advice for teenagers.

Useful websites

www.brook.org.uk Details of Brook's services, FAQs and advice for young people on contraception, sexually transmitted infections and unwanted pregnancy. Details of how to get in touch with local Brook Centre.

5

The impact of teenage sexuality on the family

In this chapter, I want to consider how the awakening sexuality of a teenager affects the family. It is probably true to say that, of all adolescent behaviour, early sexuality poses more of a challenge for parents than anything else. There are at least two reasons for this. On the one hand, the sexuality of a young person in a family has a subtle but powerful impact on the sexuality of the adults. The wishes, fears, inhibitions and needs of adults are inevitably heightened by the fact that a child in the family is taking the first steps towards sexual maturity.

On the other hand, it is often through sexual expression that the teenager most clearly challenges adult values and adult authority. If parents can understand something of what the young person is experiencing at this time, the potential for conflict and difficulty will be lessened.

Let us look now at some of the issues involved, including:

The parents' own sexuality

Boundaries and limits

Sexual activity in the home
Unsuitable relationships
Lone parents
Step-families

The parent's own sexuality

I have already mentioned the fact that both children and adolescents are affected by, and learn from, the sexual behaviour of their parents. As boys and girls grow and develop, they gradually move closer to solving the puzzle of sex. One element of this search is the child's interest in love. What is love? How do two people love each other? What do two people do together if they love each other? These are not questions that are usually asked openly by children, but it is not difficult to see how questions such as these may underlie much of the curiosity that is a natural part of growing up.

If we now turn to the issue of how children get answers to these questions, it becomes immediately apparent that children's relationships with their parents are critical here. It is through observing her or his parents that a child first begins to get some clues to these central questions. These clues will be to do with physical contact, including touching and kissing, sleeping arrangements, the way the couple talk to each other, whether they want to spend time alone together and so on. The first and most influential model of love must originate from the parents' relationship.

Your child's early questions and concerns will be innocent, in the sense that they may not yet be directly connected to issues of sexual intercourse. However, as your child grows up, questions to do with babies, or the facts of life, start to become important, and so the child will be paying more attention to your own sexuality. We cannot underestimate the importance of the role played by the parents or carers in providing some of the answers to the question 'What is the meaning of sex?' Of course, many other learning experiences contribute. As the girl or boy moves through late childhood and early adolescence, he or she will be looking outward from the family, seeking answers in the families of friends, neighbours, relatives and in the media. Nonetheless, the sexuality of our parents represents a keystone in the development of each of us.

This may seem strange when we think about how young people actually behave in relation to their parents' sexual behaviour. The fact is that young people do find it quite disgusting, indeed revolting, to think about their parents making love. Why should this be so?

The strength of feeling should give us a clue. When people feel so strongly about something that they want to shut it out, or pretend it doesn't exist, this often means quite the opposite. If people want to deny something so strongly, it may be the case that they do really want to know about it, or even be part of it, but that it is too powerful or worrying for them to face up to.

All that I have been saying about the importance of the parents' sexual relationship reflects this. To a child, it is something so central, so significant, something so connected with envy and jealousy, that it is almost too much to bear. The teenager defends against this by pushing it away – by saying 'This is too horrible and disgusting to even think about'. As one 16-year-old said in a well-known TV soap, when told that her mother was pregnant 'God! How horrible! I didn't think you two even did that sort of thing anymore.'

I know that she's aware about sexual relationships between my husband and me because she has made complaints about being kept awake at night. I remember when she was 11 or 12 she overheard us making love one night, and it really upset her, really really upset her. Actually, I haven't talked about this with her for a while now, but she was absolutely disgusted. She thought that, well first of all she thought that something very unpleasant was happening, and she thought I was in pain and then when she realised that I wasn't she thought that I was absolutely disgusting, and in fact she called me a whore, and she didn't want to have anything to do with me, and she couldn't speak to me for a few days. I mean it was really traumatic for her.

Mother of two daughters

Another important issue here has to do with the parents' relationship, and how it is affected by the young person's sexuality. I have already referred to this briefly. By the time this happens in the life of a family, the parents may have been together for 15 or 20 years. By this time, the passion of the first years will have given way to something quite different. In some cases, sex may have ceased altogether, while in others it may be an infrequent Saturday night occurrence. Some couples do maintain a satisfying sex life through a long marriage or partnership. Research shows, however, that these couples are in a minority.

As a result of this, it may well be that the subject of sexuality is a difficult one in the family. If one or other partner feels unfulfilled, and has sexual needs that are not being met, this may cause stress or conflict. Some people find that the gradually lessening sexual activity that comes with age is a frightening reminder of the failing body. All sorts of emotional issues within the partnership may affect the amount of sex that takes place. For example, anger or depression are two things which hinder the expression of loving feelings, and therefore get in the way of a satisfying sex life.

All this is important because, if sex is a difficult subject between the couple, then the teenager's sexual activity is going to be that much more tricky to deal with. Without realising it, parents or carers may feel jealous or envious of their teenager. It is certainly hard to find that your daughter or son is having a passionate sexual relationship, when your own sex life is virtually non-existent. Alternatively, it may be that parents whose own sexual needs are unfulfilled will try and seek vicarious sexual gratification through the sex life of their children. There are adults who encourage early sexual activity, and enjoy hearing about every detail of the teenager's experiences. This is understandable, but it is something that parents and carers need to watch very carefully.

It is not easy to adjust to the fact that your child has grown up to the extent that she or he is a sexual being. Indeed, parents probably have as much difficulty with this idea as teenagers do when they think about their mother and father making love. All this is relevant because of the impact it has on the sort of communication that takes place. The hang-ups, the raw feelings that adults have about sex, influence the way they talk to their teenage children. To be aware of this is essential if parents and carers are to be able to provide any real assistance and support.

Boundaries and limits

Each family establishes its own boundaries in relation to sexual behaviour. From when the first baby is born the couple gradually establishes how the family deals with things like nudity, sharing the parents' bed, touching the genitals and so on. These boundaries are significant, in that they are part of the unspoken learning that takes place on matters relating to sexuality.

The families' boundaries come into new focus as the first child reaches puberty. It is at this time that changes need to occur about the way the bathroom is used, about walking around with nothing on, even about the way people touch each other. When my own two daughters reached early adolescence I was surprised at how sensitive I became about my own body. Once my daughters reached puberty I found that I did not want to be seen naked. Somehow, it seemed like an invasion of *their* privacy. I also became very careful about hugs and goodnight kisses. Suddenly, I was aware that there were two growing women in the family – not two little girls!

These things will be experienced differently in each family. Nonetheless, much of what you have long taken for granted does have to be re-examined as your children enter adolescence. Nudity, for example, now has a quite different meaning. During childhood, the fact that members of the family are able to walk around with no clothes on means:

- openness;
- trust;
- freedom;
- a family with no secrets.

Once a girl or boy becomes a teenager, nudity can represent something quite different, something not so positive. It can mean:

- no privacy;
- secrets that the teenager does not want to know about;
- a lack of freedom.

Parents need to be sensitive to these sorts of things. They also need to be sensitive to the effect of their sexual behaviour on the young person. Just as young people want privacy, they also want their parents to be private too. This becomes especially tricky as far as the parents' sexual activity is concerned.

When children are young, and they go to bed early, the later part of the evening is a time when parents can be alone. As children grow older, they stay up later. Indeed, most families reach a stage when the teenager goes to bed after the adults. For many couples, this may have the effect of reducing their private time to zero.

There may not be any time when parents can be confident that they will not be interrupted – except perhaps in the early morning. This makes it particularly important that boundaries are respected. Adults can, for example, take care to see that their bedroom door is closed, they can take care to see that the teenager will not have to listen to them having sex and so on. We expect young people to respect us. They will be more likely to do so if we make it clear that we respect their feelings too.

Sex in the home

How should parents deal with the question of whether to permit teenagers to have sex at home? For many, this seems like a really difficult issue. It is something that stirs up all sorts of contradictory feelings, and appears very tricky to resolve. Perhaps you want to say no, but can't work out quite why you have such a powerful reaction. Perhaps you want to say yes, but feel that others (your own parents, for example) will be critical of such a decision. It may be helpful if I set out the arguments on both sides.

First, let's look at the reasons parents might have for forbidding the teenager to have sex in the home:

- you will be condoning teenage sex;
- it makes you feel awkward and uncomfortable;
- it could set a bad example to younger brothers or sisters;
- it could leave the parent or carer open to criticism by neighbours, relatives or close friends.

What about some of the arguments on the other side?

- to say yes implies trust and respect of the young person;
- to say yes acknowledges that the teenager is grown up enough to have a sexual relationship;
- it makes it possible for you as a parent or carer to keep in touch with how the relationship is going;
- it gives you a chance to get to know your daughter's/ son's partner;
- it ensures that they will have sex in a comfortable, protected place, where they will be more likely to use a contraceptive. If they are doing it in the back of a car, or out in the countryside, or at someone else's house, then there is less of a chance that they will have safe sex.

Of course, there will be many factors influencing the decision. In the end, all families have to weigh up their beliefs and feelings, and take into account all the circumstances. I hope that the list of possible reasons for and against will prove helpful. To my mind, it is the final point that tips the balance. As parents, we do have responsibilities to assist young people in every possible way to protect themselves against risk. What we want least of all is an unwanted pregnancy, or a case of gonorrhoea or herpes. That is the consideration which must, surely, take precedence over all others.

With my daughter I discovered that she was sleeping with her partner in our home. I probably wished it was otherwise, but I suppose, being a pragmatist, as it was obviously already happening, there didn't really seem much point in saying you'd better go and do it elsewhere. Because I don't know where they would have gone. In the garden, or behind the bus shelter ... I don't know. So I felt uneasy in the early years because my daughter, well she wasn't 16, and I suppose there was that whole bit about should I be encouraging it or not. But again I knew there was nothing I could do. She wasn't going to stop once she'd started. Having the boy in the house was difficult. Perhaps I didn't want to have to bump into him the next morning in the kitchen. He used to leave in the early hours of the morning. We all knew what was going on. Afterwards, it was different because she had a more steady relationship, and he did used to stay and he'd be around the next day. It's partly to do with the age with me at which it felt comfortable and OK. After a couple of years with my daughter, I breathed a huge sigh of relief and

thought 'It's alright now, because she's 17 and it feels OK now.'
                    Mother of two sons and one daughter

Having said all this, if you do come to a decision that sex in your home is acceptable, the matter should not end there. There are still many issues concerning how your teenager and his/her partner behave. Most important of all is the fact that you – as parent or carer – have probably made compromises in order to come to this decision. It follows that the young people involved should, for their part, show some respect for the other members of your family. Teenagers too need to make compromises:

- they need to be considerate of younger children;
- they should be sure they don't intrude on others by playing loud music, etc;
- they should not disturb other people's sleep;
- they should be tactful and discreet, and be respectful of the privacy of others. After all they will certainly expect some privacy themselves.

Unsuitable relationships

The question of what is an unsuitable relationship is not an easy one. Parents or carers may consider someone unsuitable for a host of different reasons. At one extreme, it may just be that you are not keen on a particular girl or boy. They may be shy or awkward, they may come from a different background, they may have green hair or a tattoo, or they may simply not be 'your type of person'.

At the other extreme, there may be an objective reason for your concern – the individual may be using drugs, or may be 10 years older than your son or daughter:

> *Well, I suppose you just have to find out about it for yourself by doing it. I mean I did, we all did, you've got to make your own mistakes, you can't say to somebody 'Don't do that because it's gonna hurt you, you're gonna end up really unhappy if you do that'. It's unreal, you know you did exactly the same thing and it was the wrong thing to do but you can't live somebody else's life for them by saying 'That would be a mistake'. OK, you might try to stop someone doing something that would physically hurt them, or you know, you're not gonna let them go off and kill themselves, but as far as the emotions are concerned you've got to go through it, you just have to.*
>
> Mother of one daughter

Parents and carers are faced with an awkward dilemma. If they express their disapproval, it is hardly likely to go down well with their teenager. On the other hand, to keep quiet and say nothing can be very hard indeed. As in the previous section, I am going to tackle this issue by looking at some of the arguments for and against telling your daughter or son what you really think. The reasons for being open and frank are:

- you are being honest;
- to say what you think may make you feel better;
- you believe you are trying to protect your teenager from the hurt that may be caused by an unsuitable relationship.

The reasons against being open and frank are as follows:

- you may force the teenager further into the arms of the unsuitable partner;
- relationships between you and your teenager may deteriorate as a result of your honesty;
- you may be imposing your standards or your preferences on your teenager.

How can parents deal with this? There are some things which are important to keep in mind.

Parents need to accept that their likes and dislikes may not be the same as the likes and dislikes of their teenager

This may be hard to swallow, but it is a fact of life. You don't expect your teenager to like all your friends. Why should they? They didn't choose them. So, in exactly the same way, there is no compelling reason why you should like the people they are keen on. Allowing young people to grow up and make their own choices in life – in friends and in sexual partners, as in other things – is part of the challenge of being a parent.

Rejecting your daughter or son's lover may be interpreted as a rejection of them too

Young people in early relationships are especially sensitive to how their parents react. They themselves are not sure if they are making the right choice. This may make them defensive. It also makes it difficult for them to listen to any criticism of their partner. Thus a parent who expresses doubts about a teenager's sexual partner will be expressing doubts about the teenager's wisdom and maturity.

What can we conclude from all this? If at all possible, parents should resist the temptation to be frank and honest. Teenagers are bound to make some mistakes in their first relationships. These mistakes are essential – in fact, they are part of the learning process. This is the way young people sort out – sometimes painfully and slowly – who they want to live with. Parents need to allow some leeway. Someone once said that teenagers are 'apprentice adults'. This is a good phrase, and reminds us that apprentices do not always get everything right at the beginning. There are bound to be mistakes, and some of those mistakes will be sexual ones.

Nonetheless, all parents have limits and boundaries, and there may be situations which are intolerable. I mentioned drugs as one of these possibilities. If, for example, your son or daughter gets involved with someone who is using drugs in a serious way, then you will be faced with a cruel dilemma. All the issues raised earlier still apply, but, in addition, there will be your fears about the effect on your teenager of being encouraged into a lifestyle that poses significant risks.

Not all families deal with such a situation in the same way. It is worth remembering, however, that you have a right to express your concerns about the health and safety of your teenager. In addition, teenagers need their parents to share with them, at an appropriate time, their values and beliefs. They also need their parents to tell them where the limits are. This may sometimes be counter-productive, leading to a wider rift in the family. More often, however, the young person feels relief that someone has laid down some guidelines. By using these guidelines, the young person may find the strength to move back towards safer, less risky behaviour.

Lone parents

Bringing up teenagers on your own is bound to create a range of stresses and difficulties. Some lone parents may have experienced an unhappy divorce or separation. Others may be adjusting to the death of a loved partner. What is certainly true is that lone parents have many needs, some of which will be different from those living in couple families. This is not the place to enter into a lengthy discussion about lone parenthood. Further reading is suggested at the end of the chapter. There are, however, particular issues concerning sexuality that I will mention briefly here.

Lone parents can find themselves both lonely and desperately missing the absent partner. As a result of this, a parent on their own is likely to experience, at some time or another, sadness, depression and a sense of emptiness. Much of this will be emotional, but such feelings are bound to have an effect on sexual need, and may lead to behaviour which affects a teenage daughter or son. It is worthwhile for lone parents to keep in mind the fact that adolescents in the family have needs too. All members of the family will have difficulty in adjusting to a complex situation. The following ideas may prove helpful.

Don't compete sexually

The fact that a lone parent becomes sexually available means that she or he may be looking for a partner. This may be exactly what the young person is doing. It could be the case, therefore, that in the same family two generations are struggling with the same issues of dating, making themselves attractive, worrying about their eligibility and so on. In such situations, a sense of competition may be created, which is the last thing that young people need. After all, for a young person, a parent is a source of support and information, as well as someone who can set the limits. If you are a rival to your teenager in the sexual success stakes you will find it that much more difficult to fill the parental role.

Don't flaunt your sexuality

We have already referred to the difficulty young people have in accepting, or even thinking about, their parents as sexual beings. It is not easy, therefore, for teenagers to be brought face to face with a parent flirting, cuddling, kissing or showing other signs of being involved in a sexual relationship. Parents should be discreet, if this is at all possible. Your teenager needs privacy, but he or she also needs you to keep some aspects of your life private too. Your sexual behaviour falls squarely into this category.

Maintain appropriate boundaries

This is probably the hardest thing of all for parents to do if they are feeling vulnerable and alone. The teenager will only too easily slip into the role of companion and confidante. This is seductive for the young person, as well as providing much needed emotional support for the adult. Parents should, however, think very carefully about the demands they make on their teenage children in such situations. Where boundaries become blurred, the teenager may:

- become over-involved;
- obtain too much gratification from meeting the needs of the adult;
- be hindered from making appropriate same-age relationships;
- feel trapped by the parent's dependence.

All this is to be avoided. It is always difficult to balance up the differing needs of each member of a family. Adults, however, should keep in mind that they have a role and a responsibility as parents or carers. The role involves keeping some distance and some detachment from the young person. The responsibility involves ensuring that teenagers are free to move gradually away from their parents in order to seek relationships outside the home:

Moodiness and temper, and I mean, that's always been a problem with us throughout her life. I mean maybe it's a case of being a single parent, it's a very intense relationship. I mean it's always very fraught for most people, I'm sure, all other single parents I know have had similar sorts of problems. But she, she was always a very wilful child, and so it was always sort of tantrums and screams, and there were certainly points when I would have given her away to anyone who would have taken her. We had terrible, terrible rows, we used to scream and shout at each other. And you know as she got older there was just an awful lot of this sort of bickering and bitching and sniping at each other. Afterwards I would think, you know, 'why on earth don't I just let it go and ignore it?' I'm drawn into her moods, you know, and I always got wound up by it. I didn't really learn how to deal with it properly. I just used to end up

time after time sort of sitting in a fume and thinking
'why did I let myself get wound up again?'
                        Mother of one daughter

Step-families

There are particular reasons why sexuality in step-families needs attention. These issues are not necessarily different from those in other types of families, but because of the strong emotions and fragile relationships, sexuality sometimes becomes more overtly important.

We have already noted that all teenagers have some difficulty in accepting their parents' sexuality. Most young people prefer not to think about this subject. In the step-family situation, especially if a parent falls in love and remarries, the children are brought face to face with the parent as a sexually active individual. Young people may find this very hard to cope with. The un-usually strong feelings that are created by the sexual be-haviour of the adult may lead the teenager to act in a strange or puzzling manner. If you notice the young person behaving oddly, ask yourself whether your sexuality has anything to do with it. Some teenagers may want to change bedrooms (so as not to hear what is going on at night). Some may refuse to go to bed until hours after the parents are asleep. Others may refuse to go on outings or take part in activities when the two adults are likely to be together. Others may act out, or draw attention to themselves in some inappropriate way, when there is any physical contact between husband and wife. These reactions may appear unnecessary, or even extreme, but for some teenagers the sexual relationship between parent and step-parent seems at times literally unbearable.

Jealousy is a major issue in all step-families. Clearly jealousy and sexuality are closely linked. If feelings of jealousy already exist, then evidence of sexuality just makes things worse, because it emphasises the closeness and intimacy between the new couple. It may also be true that an obviously sexual relationship between a parent and a 'stranger' can lead to feelings of jealousy in the teenager, sometimes to a quite unexpected extent.

Another dimension to this subject is the possibility of sexual feelings between adults and teenagers. In intact families, where the parents have seen the children grow up from babyhood onwards, sexual feelings are usually taboo. However, the situation in step-families may be more difficult. This is because the step-parent may only come to know the teenager once she or he is sexually mature. The possibility that a step-parent will feel sexually attracted to a young person cannot be ignored, and such circumstances need to be very carefully managed. Where feelings of jealousy already exist, a sense of rivalry may develop between the teenager and his or her natural parent. This can, in turn, lead to the possibility that sexuality will be used as a weapon in a family struggle for love and attention.

If a step-parent does feel sexually attracted to a stepson or stepdaughter he or she should not express these feelings, and should not allow them to develop. If at all possible, this should be discussed with the natural parent. If the feelings continue, it would be wise to seek professional help. It may be necessary for the two people to spend as little time as possible with each other. In some situations, the boy or girl may need to live away from home for a while. It is essential to be clear that these feelings must not be allowed to develop. I discuss some of these issues further in Chapter 8.

So far, I have talked about the feelings that adults may have for a stepson or stepdaughter, but the opposite situation can also arise. It may happen that a teenager becomes sexually attracted to a step-parent, and this too can create difficult circumstances. Adults do need to be aware of how they may affect young people. This is especially so at a time of life when teenagers can be impressionable, and responsive to the affection of an older person who is in an important position in the family.

Many of the things that I have discussed in this chapter apply to all families, not just to step-families. However, because of the sensitivities involved, it is particularly crucial that step-parents maintain boundaries, and recognise the power of sexual feelings in new family situations.

Here are some guidelines for step-parents that may prove helpful:

- Don't behave in any way that could be seen by the teenager as sexually provocative or suggestive.
- Don't walk around the house with nothing on.
- Don't dress or undress where you might be seen by a young person.
- Do keep the bathroom and bedroom door closed. Make it clear to teenagers in the family that you expect the same from them.
- Do maintain your own privacy with your partner. It is not necessary to kiss or cuddle in front of young people. If you are having a passionate sexual relationship, do be discreet, and remember the sensibilities of other members of the family.
- Do not intrude on the privacy of the teenager. Privacy is extremely important to a young person, especially in a step-family.

Useful organisations

Gingerbread is an organisation which provides support, help and social activities for lone parents and their children. It lists support groups, publications and has a free helpline. Contact them at 7 Sovereign Court, Sovereign Close, London E1W 3HW. Tel: 0800 018 4318. Email: office@gingerbread.org.uk

Parentline offers help and advice to parents on all aspects of bringing up young people. Their free telephone helpline is: 0808 800 2222.

Parents Advice Centre offers a variety of services to parents of teenagers. Contact their head office at Floor 4, Franklin House, 12 Brunswick Street, Belfast, BT2 7GE. Tel: (028) 9023 8800 (helpline). Email: belfast@pachelp.org

National Family and Parenting Institute supports parents and families by providing information, advice and publications. Contact them at 430 Highgate Studios, 53–79 Highgate Road, London NW5 1TL. Tel: 020 7424 3460. Email: info@nfpi.org

Useful reading

The Pill by John Guillebaud – Oxford University Press (1997). Comprehensive handbook which presents the facts, dispels the myths and answers the most commonly asked questions about oral contraceptives.

Contraception – A User's Handbook by Anne Szarewski – Oxford University Press (2000). Provides up-to-the-minute information and clear and reliable advice.

Useful websites

www.gingerbread.org.uk lists the organisation's services and network of support groups.

www.fpa.org.uk provides information about contraception, sexual health, publications and resources for young people, parents and professionals.

www.parentsadvicecentre.org provides information about its services to families under stress.

www.nfpi.org.uk promotes the work of the National Family and Parenting Institute.

www.e-parents.org a website set up by the National Family and Parenting Institute which has information, advice and up-to-date news about all aspects of parenting and families.

6

Risky behaviour

To take risks often seems to be a natural part of adolescent behaviour. To experiment, to test the boundaries, to sail as close to the wind as possible – all this may seem inevitable with teenagers. In fact, as we shall see, there are wide differences between individuals, and many young people remain cautious and conservative in their behaviour. Nonetheless, it is important to understand what underlies a teenager's need to take risks if we are to make sense of early sexual development. In this chapter, I will provide a background by looking at some features of adolescent development, as well as exploring some of the consequences of risk-taking.

Issues to be covered here include:

The nature of adolescence

Sexual risks

Teenage pregnancy

Sexually transmitted infections (STIs)

HIV/AIDS

Assault, rape and exposure to violence

The parents' response

The nature of adolescence

As I have already indicated, adolescence is best seen as a transitional stage. The young person moves from childhood to adulthood in a slow process. As with all transitions, the move from one stage to another causes a variety of conflicting emotions. These include:

- anxiety about the future;
- frustration at the limitations imposed by adults;
- uncertainty about when adulthood has been reached;
- loss of childhood certainties;
- hopes for success and achievement.

All these concerns lead the teenager to ask some fundamental questions. Let us look at one or two of these.

'When am I grown up?'

It is understandable that the young person wants to know when she/he will be considered to have reached adult status. The problem is that no one can give a clear answer. In our society, there are many ways of defining maturity. The law is muddled, and allows young people to do some things at 16, some at 17 and others at 18. Parents, teachers, social workers and magistrates all have a different view on this question. The result is that teenagers often get frustrated, and may decide to take things into their own hands. A young man, or young woman, may feel compelled to push the boundaries, challenging adults to see how far he or she can go.

'What can I do?'

Closely linked to this is the question of what activities are not allowed at different ages. This applies to drinking, smoking and staying out late, but it also applies to sexual behaviour. Young people need to know what they can do, and who can blame them? We all need to know what the rules are, and teenagers are no different from the rest of us (see Chapter 8 – Sex and the law).

'I want to be different'

Part of the process of growing up involves sorting out who you are. A central theme running through the adolescent stage is 'Who am I?' To answer this question, a teenager needs to feel different from his or her parents. A young person can only feel real – someone who actually exists in their own right – if he or she can be sure of being distinct. Being distinct means not being part of the parent. Psychologists use the phrase 'negative identity' to describe this stage. To paraphrase, the young person is saying 'I don't know who I am, but I do know that I am not going to be like you.' Of course, this is only a stage, and teenagers are influenced by their parents, and do take on some of their characteristics. For a period in adolescence, however, to be different is essential. It is the only way you can be sure

you are you, and not the person your parents want you to
be.

'Can I do anything at all?'

It is often said that teenagers go through a period when a
tiny part of them needs to believe that they are omni-
potent – that they can do anything at all. This is closely
linked to a belief that nothing can happen to them, that
they can handle any situation, that they are all-powerful.
Such beliefs are no doubt a defence against exactly the
opposite – feelings of intense self-doubt, and fears of not
being able to manage anything at all.

All these characteristics of adolescence are associated
with the possibility of risk-taking. You want to be grown
up, so you need to show that you can do grown-up things.
You don't want someone to tell you what to do, so you go
over the limit – just to make a point. You have to be
different from your parents – they are safe and boring, so
you are daring. You can do anything you want – nothing
can touch you. So why worry about taking precautions?

Sexual risks

All the points outlined above are relevant to sexual risk-
taking. However, in addition, there are a couple of further
things that are a part of the overall picture. The first is that
freedom can be an intoxicating experience. Some young
people may be very cautious, wanting to postpone sexual
activity until a later time, or wanting to keep it only for a
very special relationship.

However, there will be others who may get carried
away with the discovery that sex without responsibility is

wonderful. Good sexual experiences are very pleasurable indeed. It is not hard to see how in some circumstances, teenagers can get carried away with the possibility of unlimited sexual pleasure.

Closely related to this is the fact that some of us are fundamentally greedy. When faced with lots and lots of a good things – whether it's food, or drink, or sex – there are people who want as much as they can get – and more! Personality factors play a part here, but so does maturity. In order to be sensible, and to recognise that unlimited excess is not always good for us, we need self-control. The ability to exercise self-discipline comes with age, and we should perhaps not judge young people too harshly if this is a lesson they have yet to learn. Parents and other adults can help, as much by example as by anything else. If your teenager sees you grabbing the next cigarette, or the next drink, as if your life depends on it, it will be that much harder for him or her to discover their own self-control. Parents are role models in so many different ways – even where greed is concerned!

I have already mentioned a common adolescent belief that 'it can't happen to me'. This is absolutely central to the question of whether teenagers are able to avoid risky behaviour. It is often said of teenage pregnancy 'It is not a question of why a girl fails to use contraception. The question is rather – why would a young woman want to take precautions?' The implication here is that you only take precautions if:

- you are able to plan ahead;
- you have a sense of the future;
- you have a good reason for not getting pregnant – such as exams, a career, etc.;
- you have realised that you are as subject to risk as anyone else.

I believe it is helpful to put the question this way around. In particular, it encourages us not to blame teenagers for their risky behaviour. If we can focus on the fact that young people need certain characteristics to *avoid* risks, we can begin to see just how hard it is for a teenager to be sensible and grown up all the time:

> *I mean, my friend, she's 14, and as I say, you know, she lays about with anything and that. And I think it's good we learnt about sex and contraceptives and that, like, early, when we did. Because she came from my school. I don't think it's too young, because I think we need to know. I think when we get to our age anyway you get, like, sensual tendencies, and you just feel as though you need to. I think even if we hadn't had sex education when we were younger, this would have happened anyway with her, I think, like as I say at our age you just, you feel you have to experiment and that sort of thing. You have to know what life's all about. You only learn from mistakes.*
>
> 15-year-old girl

Before concluding this section, I do need to emphasise that young people vary enormously. Not all teenagers are risk-takers, and we have to be careful not to judge everyone in the same way. As with all things, so much will depend on family circumstances, on the social situation of the young person and on their individual character. While adolescence may make risk-taking behaviour more likely, this does not mean that all young people are compelled to engage in risky activities. Some tread very carefully indeed, avoiding all situations where there is any danger. Others may tentatively test out their own capacity to cope with risk, but in a limited and sensible manner. Risky behaviour is common in the teenage years. Not all teenagers, however, will be risk-takers.

Teenage pregnancy

It is now time to look at some of the things that can happen as a result of risky behaviour, turning first to teenage pregnancy. When parents and schools teach about menstruation, and about conception, they rarely give enough attention to the signs of pregnancy. Many girls fear that a late or missed period means that they are pregnant, but, of course, there can be a variety of reasons which lie behind irregularity in the menstrual cycle. All girls should know something about this. They should also know where they can go for further information, and what they can do to find out whether they are pregnant. This is the sort of basic information which no one likes to provide, because to discuss it implies that it might happen.

However, it can happen. And it does happen. Britain has very high rates of teenage pregnancy, compared with other European countries. In very approximate terms, 9 out of every 1,000 girls under the age of 16 become pregnant in our country each year. For a girl or young woman to experience an unwanted pregnancy is an extremely upsetting situation for all concerned, including the parents or carers. Neither should we forget the young man in these circumstances, who will also have major personal issues to deal with. In spite of the possible shock and distress for the parents when such an event occurs, their reaction at this point is absolutely critical.

It will have implications not only for how the situation is resolved, but also for the future relationship between the teenagers and their parents. If at all possible, adults need to stay calm. They should not overreact. If they can support their daughter or son at this point, the young person will remember it all their lives. It may seem to an adult like the end of the world. However, good advice will help everyone to see things in a different light. An unwanted pregnancy is not the end of the world, but a critical turning point in the teenager's life. The role of the parent or carer at this juncture will make all the difference.

There will be a number of options to consider. If the parent can consider these with the young person, so much the better. If not, then the adult should ensure that the girl or boy – with his or her partner – think through all the possible courses of action very carefully indeed. This is where good advice is worth its weight in gold. The names and addresses of useful organisations are listed at the end of this chapter. The teenager should be encouraged to talk to a well-trained and responsible professional who has experience in this area. The young person needs to take time to make the right decision, and will inevitably need help in this process.

Parents and carers also have to decide what they can do to help in this situation. Once the adult is clear about this, then it should be communicated to the teenager. What assistance is the parent going to offer? The young person should know where she or he stands, and what he or she can expect from the family.

Adults may have a variety of reactions. These may include:

- *Shame*. What will other people think?
- *Guilt*. Where did I go wrong?
- *Anger*. How could my son/daughter let me down like this?
- *Resentment*. How will this affect me and my life?

All these feelings are perfectly normal. Adults should take an opportunity to air their feelings with a close and trusted friend, or with a professional counsellor. This will help the parent to get things in perspective.

However strong the parent's feelings, he or she should never forget that this young person, a parent-to-be, is still a teenager. He or she needs the parent's support, especially at this moment. The importance of parental support cannot be over-estimated.

What are the options? There are essentially three:

- to have an abortion (sometimes called a termination of pregnancy);
- to continue with the pregnancy, and to have the baby;
- to have the baby, but arrange for it to be adopted at birth.

It needs to be acknowledged that every one of these options has disadvantages. To have a termination may leave the girl with a range of difficult feelings, especially of feelings of guilt and loss. Alternatively, the young woman may want to continue with the pregnancy, but this will obviously affect her education and career plans. Questions of childcare, and the future relationship with the father, need to be taken into account. Lastly, the baby could be adopted. While some do make this decision, it is not an easy one to manage. All involved should recognise that, once the baby is born, it will be very hard indeed to give it up.

Throughout this section, I have talked about the young man as well as the young woman. In thinking about teenage pregnancy, there tends to be far more of an emphasis on the young woman's situation. She, after all, is the one who will have the termination or bear the child. Nonetheless, the role of the teenage father – or potential father – does need to be highlighted. If there is a strong relationship between the young man and the young woman, it will be that much easier for everyone involved to come to the best decision. Teenage fathers too often get pushed to the margins in such situations, preventing them from contributing in the way they would wish. Furthermore, too little attention is paid to the young man's need for support and assistance. Pregnancy involves two people. There is no doubt that both will be better served if their partnership can be fully recognised by the two families concerned.

Sexually transmitted infections (STIs)

While everyone has heard of AIDS, not everyone knows that there are many other sexually transmitted infections. While these may not cause death, they can have many other unpleasant and serious health implications. Those most often seen today include chlamydia, herpes and gonorrhoea. It is worrying that, over the last 10 years, the incidence of these infections has increased markedly in the population. Most worrying of all, however, is the fact that the increases have been greater in young people than in older age groups.

Chlamydia is the most common sexually transmitted infection, although strangely it is the least well known. As a result, it is hardly ever mentioned or discussed. Rates of chlamydia infection have increased more sharply over the last decade than have rates for any other sexually transmitted infection. Chlamydia can be treated with a simple course of antibiotics, but, if left untreated, can damage the fallopian tubes in females (leading to infertility), and can cause sterility in males.

It is essential that both parents and teenagers are aware of the facts in relation to sexually transmitted infections (sometimes known as STIs). For a variety of reasons young people are especially vulnerable to the possibility of contracting an STI. Here are some possible reasons for this:

- teenagers may not wish to admit that they are sexually active;
- teenagers may find it difficult to talk about sex;
- teenagers may feel invulnerable, as if nothing can happen to them;
- teenagers often lack the confidence necessary to obtain information or to seek assistance;
- for a teenager to take precautions means that he or she must plan ahead.

There is a lot parents can do in this area. Talking about STIs is as important as talking about contraception. Adults should not avoid the subject because they fear being a scaremonger. They should be firm ('You must protect yourself'), but can also be reassuring ('You can protect yourself').

These are some of the things teenagers must know:

- anyone who is sexually active can contract an STI;
- the most common way that STIs are transmitted is through sexual intercourse;
- while AIDS may be the most dangerous STI, other STIs can have serious long-term consequences, such as infertility;
- most STIs do not have obvious symptoms;
- apart from abstinence, or only having sex with one

trusted partner, the best protection against STIs is to use a condom;
- when one person has an STI, then the partner is likely to contract it as well;
- treatment for STIs is confidential, and widely available (see end of chapter).

Anyone who has any of the following symptoms should seek treatment:

- painful burning sensations during urination, or dark-coloured urine;
- a discharge from the vagina or penis that itches, burns or has a strong smell;
- sores, redness, or irritation in the genital area;
- a persistent sore throat.

When we had a lesson in Year 12 about them (STIs), I was really quite shocked at how ignorant I was, and it wasn't just me. Talking to other people afterwards, you know, we were all, you know, very naive. Like, there were things I just didn't have a clue about. I was quite surprised at how little I did know because I thought I knew a lot more. I was just really surprised basically, and so were my friends.

18-year-old boy

HIV/AIDS

Because AIDS has received so much publicity since the mid-1980s, many people believe they know a lot about the disease. Studies show that teenagers may know more about this than about other sexual topics. Nonetheless, there is still much ignorance about the subject. In Britain, the high level of public anxiety seen in the late 1980s has given way to a different attitude. As figures in the last few years have shown relatively low levels of infection among the heterosexual population, health education campaigns have shifted in their approach. These now focus on high-risk groups such as intravenous drug users, and most teenagers have little opportunity to discuss issues to do with HIV/AIDS.

In spite of this, HIV remains the one STI that can cause death, and it cannot be ignored. This may not be so obvious in a country such as Britain, but, it is of course, a very different matter in Africa, in Russia or in the Far East. Even in Britain, there are currently in the region of 2,500 new diagnoses of HIV every year. Because of the treatment approach called 'combination therapy', which uses several different drugs together, many of those infected with the virus are now living longer and more normal lives. However, not all can benefit from combination therapy, and it remains a fact that there is still no known cure for HIV.

There are a number of things young people should know about HIV/AIDS. These are:

- HIV/AIDS is not a homosexual disease. While, in the early years, cases occurred primarily in the homosexual population, today intravenous drug users are particularly at risk, as are men and women having sex with someone who is HIV positive.
- In spite of the success of combination therapy, such treatment cannot eliminate HIV from the body. It is misleading to think that there is now a cure, or that HIV/AIDS is no longer a problem in Britain.
- The HIV virus is transmitted through bodily fluids in the male and female sexual organs, as well as through

blood. In addition to transmission through sex, an open cut or sore may be a source through which the virus can enter the body.

- Apart from abstinence from sex, the safest protection from HIV is the same as for other sexually transmitted infections, namely the use of a condom.

As with other risk factors, the more parents and carers can inform themselves about HIV/AIDS, the more likely they will be to inform their young people. Suggestions for further reading on this topic are at the end of the chapter.

Assault and exposure to violence

We have already given some thought to this issue in our discussion on personal safety in Chapter 4. As with all issues like this, it is one thing to advise a young person what to do, and it is quite another to see that they take the advice.

In the first place, it is important that the teenager, and this applies to both boys and girls, knows that there are things that he or she can do to avoid danger. These include:

- Recognising that teenagers are not invulnerable. There are circumstances that the young person will not be able to handle.
- Accepting that there are places, and situations, which are best avoided. These include city areas after dark, being alone in a car with a stranger and so on.

- Making every attempt to plan ahead. This applies to having enough money for a telephone call, taking a mobile phone, booking a taxi, finding out about public transport and so on.

The possibility of your teenager being exposed to violence is the sort of thing that parents worry about, when lying awake at 3:00 in the morning. We may fear it, yet, strangely, we do not find it easy to talk openly about it. There are a number of inhibitions which prevent us from talking sensibly about the subject of violence.

In the first place, even to raise the topic may make you sound fussy and overprotective. It is true that there are teenagers who react badly to expressions of concern about their safety. Nonetheless, parents should not be put off by this. You have a right and a responsibility to do everything you can to ensure that your son or daughter remains safe. If your teenager doesn't like it, you need to have a full and frank discussion.

Second, you may not wish to raise questions to do with danger and violence, for the same reason that you may be tempted to avoid other tricky issues. To talk about it seems to imply that it might happen. This is simply not a good reason – don't hide behind it.

Third, you may not want to discuss the topic because you don't know what the answer is. We cannot keep our children completely safe. However, there are many things we can do. These include:

- making sure that they are well informed;
- letting them know that you are concerned about their welfare;
- providing them with strategies and options which are available if they need them.

The parent's response

Let us look more closely at what parents can do. There are, in fact, two questions to consider here:

- Is there anything parents can do to prevent risky behaviour?
- What should parents do if things go wrong?

Can parents prevent risky behaviour?

The answer to this is probably not. In the end, if young people are determined to drink too much, or drive a car without a licence, or have sex behind the bike sheds without using a condom, there is not much that parents can do to stop them.

However, do remember that not all adolescents are driven to engage in risky behaviour. Many are cautious and conservative in what they do. As for those who do take risks, there are a number of things that can be done by parents and carers. These are things that will reduce the young person's need to challenge adult authority, and so help the teenager to take fewer risks. Here are some suggestions:

- *Keep in mind what it is that your teenager needs from you.* Young people respond best to parents and other adults who are firm but fair. They do not want adults to exercise the heavy hand of authority. That will just cause conflict. Neither do they want a permissive, hands-off approach. They do not want you to say 'OK, it's your life, get on with it'. This feels like a rejection. Young people need you to steer a middle course – involved and caring, but clear about what you believe in.

- *Show respect*. One of the things young people complain about most is that adults do not respect their point of view. Teenagers do have worthwhile things to say, and they should be given a chance to express their opinions. Often they have sensible suggestions to offer which parents have not even considered. If you are in a discussion or in a disagreement with your daughter or son, do give them a fair hearing. If you respect them, they are more likely to respect you, and to take seriously your point of view.

- *Be clear about what you consider acceptable*. As I have indicated in previous chapters, young people need to know where they stand. They need to know what the limits are. This doesn't mean they will always respect them. They will challenge authority, and disobey the rules as a way of showing they are grown up. Having the rules and limits is essential, however, for without them what does your teenager have to hold on to? The limits you set are the framework around which the young person constructs their own safe and sensible rules for living.

- *Be supportive*. Do make it clear that you are there if you are needed. For a teenager, one of the most re-assuring things is to know that a parent or carer will be available at times of stress or difficulty. However much anger and conflict there is, however much shouting and screaming and arguing goes on, teenagers do need their parents. That is something that no adult should ever forget.

What should parents do if things go wrong?

However difficult the situation, your response at a time of
crisis will have a profound influence on later events. A
crisis can happen in many different ways. You may be
woken up by a phone call from the police in the middle
of the night. You may be called to the headteacher's office.
You may discover a syringe under your teenager's bed. A
neighbour may tell you something about your son or
daughter which you didn't know. Your teenager may,
late at night, confide in you a worry about a sexually
transmitted infection. All these, and many other things,
are possible. What advice is there?

- *If the worst happens, try not to overreact.* However
  difficult it is, try to remain calm. You may feel distressed, furious, ashamed or guilty. Do make every
  effort to contain your feelings. To paraphrase a well-
  known saying: *'React in haste, repent at leisure'*. If you
  allow your feelings a free rein, you may very well
  regret their effect later on. I know I have said this a
  number of times already, but remember, in a time of
  crisis your teenager needs you more than at any other
  moment.
- *If you do get angry or upset, and you can't contain your
  emotions, then try and find a way of talking about how
  you feel.* Be adult yourself. Be honest, acknowledge
  how strongly you feel, but *make it clear that you are
  there to help.*
- *Be well informed.* Whatever the subject, whether it is
  drugs, pregnancy or STIs, do everything you can to
  find out about it. Learn as much as you can. This
  includes seeking out helpful organisations. The
  better informed you are, the more likely it is that the
  right decision will be taken.

- *Don't be ashamed to seek help.* Many parents find this the most difficult step to take. To look for help may feel like an admission of failure. It isn't. You will be surprised at how many other families experience similar crises and difficulties. One of the things that parents frequently say is that to learn that you are not alone, to find that others are in the same boat, can make all the difference in the world.
- *There are some situations where you need professional help.* If you feel out of your depth, or uncertain what to do next, then ask for advice. You have a responsibility to do so for the sake of your son or daughter. Helpful organisations are listed throughout this book.

Useful organisations

British Pregnancy Advisory Service – for advice on pregnancy, abortion and contraception contact: BPAS Head Office, Austy Manor, Wootton Wawen, Solihull, West Midlands B95 6BX. Actionline: 08457 304030.

Young Minds provides information and advice for anyone with concerns about the mental health of children and young people. Contact them at 102–108 Clerkenwell Road, London, EC1M 5SA. Parents Info Service: 0800 018 2138.

National AIDS helpline is a national phoneline offering confidential advice, information and referrals on any aspect of HIV/AIDS to anyone. It is open every day, 24 hours a day. Tel: 0800 567 123.

The Terrence Higgins Trust – parents or young people can contact this charity for information, advice and help on any aspect of HIV or AIDS at 52–54 Gray's Inn Road, London WC1X 8JE. Helpline: 020 7242 1010.

The Suzy Lamplugh Trust provides personal safety advice and training and produces videos and other publications. Their contact address is: 14 East Sheen Avenue, London SW14 8AS. Tel: 020 8876 0305.

Useful websites

www.bpas.org the website for the British Pregnancy Advisory Service.

www.youngminds.org.uk contains parent information service, factsheets and details of consultancy and training.

www.lovelife.hea.org.uk is a website by the Health Development Agency answering questions on STIs HIV, AIDS and sexual health matters.

www.tht.org.uk provides facts, advice, publications and services to people with or affected by HIV and people at risk.

www.suzylamplugh.org offers advice sheets, information about conferences and training courses
and lists of publications.

www.ruthinking.co.uk is a website for young
people which provides information on safer sex,
contraception, abortion and STIs.

7

Sexual orientation

The process of understanding sexual orientation

It is important to start by acknowledging that all young people, at some time or other, wonder about their sexual orientation. It is an inevitable part of growing up – a perfectly natural question to ask. It is also part of a wider search for an identity which involves the adolescent in trying to work out exactly what sort of person she or he is.

There are many components to this search. Some are to do with the sort of relationship the teenager is looking for: short term or long term; close or relatively detached; dependent or independent. Other aspects are to do with plans and goals for the future, while still others concern values and beliefs. In addition to all this, there is the question 'Am I more attracted to people of the same gender as myself, or to people of the opposite gender?'

This is a question to which there may not be an immediate answer. Although it is true that some people know from childhood or early adolescence that they are definitely gay or straight, the majority resolve this question slowly during the course of their teenage years.

Indeed, many go through what is known as a transient stage. Thus, there are teenagers who have heterosexual relationships but who, in due course, become gay or lesbian. In the same way, there are those who go through a stage of homosexuality – having a crush on someone, engaging in mutual masturbation, or experiencing a full sexual relationship – who become heterosexual adults. What is important to understand is that a period of uncertainty is a perfectly natural part of adolescent development. People do not necessarily have a clear and definite answer to their sexual orientation. They may need a number of different experiences, with different sorts of people, before they can be confident about whether they are heterosexual or homosexual:

> *I suppose I started to have sexual feelings – I didn't categorise them in any way – from the age of 11, I suppose, and those feelings carried on until I was 14, 15. It was only then through watching tele-vision, talking to friends, that I would probably categorise some of them, not all of them, as gay thoughts. The actual process of realising that I was one of those 'poof' things that everybody had been talking about at school, was a very long process. It didn't really finish if you like until I was 16, maybe 17. Very late on, really. I just thought that they were ordinary sexual feelings, which in fact they are. It's just that through images and things in the media and social pressures, our sexual feelings get channelled in one direction or the other, and in mainstream society one of those sexual feelings is good and okay and normal, and the other types are bad and to be got rid of and evil.*

> 20-year-old man

In spite of the fact that people know more about homo-sexuality today, and in spite of considerable changes, both in the law and in attitudes, there is still a large amount of ignorance about what it means to be gay or lesbian. Such ignorance has an enormous impact on young people, especially on those who are struggling with queries and uncertainties about their sexual orientation. It is impor-tant to emphasise that it is not abnormal to be gay or lesbian. People who are gay or lesbian are in the minority in our society, but they should not be judged or discrimin-ated against. This needs to be said because, sadly, there is still widespread prejudice against homosexuality.

Prejudice and misunderstanding create a situation in which it is exceptionally difficult for a teenager – indeed for anyone – to be open and honest about the fact that they may be gay or lesbian. Fears about the reactions of friends and family mean that most keep quiet. Teenagers in this situation cannot ask for help, and hardly any support is provided in schools or colleges. Young people who are gay or lesbian may have to cope with a variety of issues – at school, at work or in the family – without being able to obtain the assistance that is normally available to others of the same age.

Finding out that your teenager is gay or lesbian

One of the hardest things for any gay or lesbian young person to do is to tell their parents about their sexual preference. Most teenagers worry for a long time about how and when to discuss the matter. They will almost

certainly expect their parents to be upset, or even horri-
fied. All those who are gay or lesbian remember this
moment as a very important one in their lives. The reaction of the parents or carers is critical, for it reflects the
answer to the question all young people ask: 'Am I still
going to be loved and accepted by my family once they
know about my sexual orientation?'

Why do parents react so strongly? One obvious reason
is that adults worry about the prejudice and intolerance
that we have already discussed. This prejudice may result
in the young person facing difficulties at college or at
work, or among the peer group. Another reason relates
to having children. Generally, parents want their children
to become parents too. This may be:

- because they want to become grandparents;
- because they want the family name to continue;
- because they have invested so much in parenthood
  themselves.

Of course, there are a number of other reasons for worrying about our children's sexual orientation. These may be
less obvious, but involve strong and complicated emotions. Parents want their children to fit in, and to be the
same as everyone else. Perhaps most importantly, in some
primitive way, we want our children to be the same as us.
All of us have to come to terms with the fact that our son
or daughter is an individual. This means that he or she is
different – this is something we cannot escape. Deep
down, however, we have a sense that our children are a
part of us, a part of our identity. Their sexual preference
tells us something about their sameness or difference. To
find that a teenager is gay or lesbian means that they are as
different sexually from a heterosexual parent as they could
possibly be:

When I was 15, I started going to gay pubs and everything which you shouldn't do at that age but it's quite an awful age and I successfully managed to go out for two years until I was 17. It got to a point where I was lying about everything I did, in the family I was lying, and I just got fed up with it. So I just came out with it one night. It always comes out like one big thing. When I told my dad he was in bed at the time and I sat on the end of the bed and I said 'I'm gay'. I just watched the colour drain out of his face. It was OK to start off with but then he spoke to my mum and my mum was really upset about it. I'd sort of led them on let-ting them think I had a girl-friend and this and that. That's why they never had any idea at all. It was round about Christmas last year, and it ruined their Christmas, don't know about mine.

19-year-old man

When parents first find out that their son is gay or that their daughter is lesbian, they may well be very distressed. Some may be furious, forbidding their teenager to have anything more to do with homosexual friends. Some may get extremely upset, torturing themselves with guilt about where they went wrong. Others may refuse to discuss the situation, hoping that if they close their eyes, the whole thing will go away. All these reactions are understandable, but none will make for good relationships with your son or daughter. Let us look at some of the things that parents or carers can do when faced with this situation.

Recognise that this is not the end of the world

It is not easy for parents or carers to adjust to the discovery that their teenager is homosexual. Nonetheless, accepting the reality is essential if you are going to be able to continue to communicate with your daughter or son. At first, it may seem like a terrible blow. People describe themselves as being 'quite shattered' by the news. However, being gay or lesbian does not make the individual someone quite different. The young person is just the same as they were before they told you the news. So remember, this is not the end of the world. Rather, it is the start of a new, more honest and open relationship with your child.

Reassure your daughter or son that you still love them

As I have already indicated, the reason that young people have so much difficulty in telling their parents that they are gay or lesbian is that they fear rejection. They fear that their mother or father will turn them out of the house, or refuse to go on supporting them. What young people need in this situation – more than anything else – is to know that their parents still accept them, and will continue to care for them. Indeed, young people who are gay or lesbian need more support than others, not less. Parents do have a big responsibility here:

> *Parents should not give an immediate reaction, because immediate reactions hurt so much. Because it's taken that child so much courage to actually say something. So just think about what you are saying and go away and think about it. Think about your priorities and if you love that child more than you hate their sexuality. I think you need a lot of time to think.*
>
> 17-year-old girl

One last point. If you feel like rejecting your son or daughter because of their sexual orientation, think again. A serious rift created at the time you first learn about your son's or daughter's homosexuality will take a long time to heal. In families where this does happen, it is all too often the parents who live to regret their actions. The experience of losing a child in this way can be very painful indeed.

Ask to meet your son's or daughter's partner

One clear sign that parents can give to show that they have accepted the sexuality of the young person is to offer to meet the partner. This may not always be appropriate, since obviously in some cases there will not be a serious or steady partner to meet. Nonetheless, in situations where your daughter or son is having a relationship with someone who is special to them, then to welcome this person into your home can seem like a huge step towards acceptance and reconciliation. It may not be easy. You may have all sorts of fears and anxieties. Remind yourself that coming to terms with it all will take time. Meeting your son's or daughter's partner will send a message that you are willing to accept who they are:

> So he sat down and he said 'I've got something to tell you, and it is important' so I said 'alright, what is it?' and he said 'well, two of your old friends would understand'. And then it suddenly dawned on me which two friends he meant. And it was the gay friends we had. And I just said 'oh, so you think you are' and I didn't use the word. And he said 'yes' so I said 'well, what makes you think that?', and he said 'I just know'. So I said 'OK, you

*know, that's OK' and I could see the relief in his face,
and his absolute relief in the whole body. And I just
went up to him, and he burst into tears. I put my arms
around him and said 'that's alright, don't worry
about it'. I said 'I still love you, you're my son and
nothing's going to make any difference to the way I
feel about you. You're no different now than a minute
before you told me, so it's alright, don't worry'.*

Mother of two boys

Useful organisations

London Lesbian and Gay Switchboard
provide a 24-hour confidential advice and information service about all aspects of homosexuality.
They have information on local groups around the
country. Their address is: LLGS, PO Box 7324,
London N1 9QSA. Parents are also welcome to
phone. Tel: 020 7837 7324.

Parent's Friend is a national helpline also providing publications, including an information
pack for parents. Write for details to: Voluntary
Action Leeds, Stringer House, 34 Lupton Street,
Hunslet, Leeds LS10 2QW. Tel: 01902 820 497
for information about opening times of helpline.

Acceptance is a helpline and support group for
parents of lesbians and gay men. Their address is:
64 Holmside Avenue, Halfway Houses, Sheerness
ME12 3EY. Tel: 01795 661 463.

Families and Friends of Lesbians and Gays (FFLAG) is a national organisation with telephone helplines across the UK and parents' groups which hold regular meetings. It aims to support parents and their lesbian, gay and bisexual sons and daughters. Their address is: FFLAG, PO Box 153, Manchester, M60 1LP. Central helpline: 01454 852 418.

Useful reading

A Stranger in the Family – How to Cope if Your Child is Gay by Terry Sanderson – The Other Way Press (1996). Written by an experienced counsellor, this book provides information, support and practical advice.

There Must be Fifty Ways to Tell Your Mother by Lynn Sutcliffe – Cassell, London (1995). Personal stories, experiences and ideas from children and their parents.

Useful websites

www.llgs.org.uk provides information about the London Lesbian and Gay Switchboard services and local groups.

8

Sex and the law

There are a number of ways in which the laws concerning sexual behaviour affect young people. It is particularly important to consider these laws, since there is widespread ignorance about them among young people. To take one example, there is general confusion among 14-, 15- and 16-year-olds about medical confidentiality, and about their rights in relation to sexual health consultations.

In this chapter, I consider:

The age of consent

Confidentiality

Sexual abuse

The age of consent

The law protects children until they are old enough to make their own decisions about sex. The age at which a young person is considered old enough to make these decisions is called the age of consent. If a man or boy has sex with a girl who is below the age of consent, this person is committing an offence. In England, Scotland and Wales the age of consent is 16, although in Northern Ireland it is 17, and in the Republic of Ireland it is 18. In some European countries, it has been reduced in recent years, and it can be as low as 12, as it is now in Holland. This law does not apply to women. A girl or woman cannot be prosecuted for unlawful sexual intercourse if she has sex with a boy of any age, even someone under 16. However, there is a possibility that the woman could be prosecuted for indecent assault if the boy was under 16, although such a prosecution is very unusual.

It has to be said that many young people do have sexual relationships when either or both partners are under 16, without realising they are breaking the law. It is rare for the police to interfere, except in special circumstances. This could be because a parent or carer objects to the relationship, or it could be that a social worker believes the young person is in 'moral danger'. The grounds of 'moral danger' are sometimes used to take teenagers into care, if it is thought they are being promiscuous, or if they are involved in prostitution.

The age of consent is now 16 for both heterosexual and homosexual relationships. Until the year 2000, the homosexual age of consent was 18, but after a considerable political battle the homosexual age of consent was lowered to 16 as part of the Sexual Offences (Amendment) Act 2000. One issue which was of great concern to those who opposed the lowering of the age of homosexual consent was that of abuse of trust. These politicians were anxious that young men under the age of 18, especially immature young men, might become more vulnerable because of this change in the law. As a result, the Act incorporated a clause making it an offence for a person over the age of 18 to have a sexual relationship with a person under that age when they are deemed to be in a position of trust.

Confidentiality

Medical confidentiality is a difficult issue, and one which the law has not found easy to resolve. It should first be noted that anyone aged 16 or above has a right to confidential medical treatment. At that age, parents no longer have any legal status, in that they cannot insist on being involved or consulted about their daughter's or son's treatment.

The problem arises if the teenager is under the age of 16. The issue first came to prominence as a result of a court case brought by a Mrs Gillick against her local health authority in 1984. She wanted an assurance from the health authority that she would be consulted if a daughter of hers under the age of 16 sought contraceptive advice. The health authority refused to give such an assurance, and in the end the case went all the way to the House of Lords.

The Law Lords ruled against Mrs Gillick, arguing that in certain circumstances a young person under the age of 16 should have the right to confidential medical treatment. Such circumstances would be:

- where the girl (although under 16) will understand the doctor's advice;
- where the doctor has tried, but cannot persuade the girl to inform her parents, nor is able to persuade the girl to allow him/her to inform her parents;

- where the doctor believes that it is in the girl's best interest that the treatment be given, even though the parents have not been informed.

As a result of this case, the Department of Health issued guidelines for doctors about this issue in 1986, and in essence the position has remained the same since then. The guidelines state that a young person of any age is entitled to a confidential consultation with a doctor, provided that the young person makes it clear that she/he does not want the parents to be informed. However, a doctor who is unwilling to accept a request for confidentiality can refuse to continue with the consultation.

This has given rise to an unsatisfactory state of affairs, in that a young person has first to establish what the doctor's view about confidentiality is before knowing what she/he can expect. In practice, doctors vary widely in their beliefs about confidentiality, and it is not surprising that young people are confused. If a young person needs a confidential consultation concerning a sexual health matter, and discovers that her/his doctor will not guarantee this, then she/he is best advised to seek help from a Brook Advisory Centre or other local family planning centre.

Sexual abuse

This is the sort of subject no one likes to think about. Yet, we know that substantial numbers of children and young people are sexually abused each year. All parents and carers should be aware of the problem, and should learn something about the circumstances surrounding sexual abuse. This is especially true if the adult is also a teacher or youth worker, or is someone who comes into contact with young people in their work.

It is important not to oversimplify, since every individual circumstance will be different, and any guidelines there are can only be of the most general sort. It needs to be absolutely clear, however, that:

- incest – a sexual relationship with a close relative – is a criminal act against the child or young person;
- sexual assault is also a criminal act against the child or young person;
- sexual intercourse or any other kind of sexual intimacy by an adult with someone under 16 is an offence against the young person and can lead to prosecution. This also now applies to a homosexual act with someone under the age of 18, if the adult is in a position of trust.

Sometimes, it is hard for adults to believe that someone they know has been sexually abusing a young person. This can mean that the honesty of the child or teenager is doubted by those around them. If you are in this situation, remember that it is not easy to make up a story about sexual abuse. It is highly likely that what you are hearing is the truth.

It is often believed that, so long as the actual abuse can be prevented from occurring again, the whole matter is best forgotten. Sadly this is not the case, since adults who sexually abuse young people may be unable to stop, and may well go on to abuse other children in the family, or others whom they know well. Also the young person who has been abused will need help to undo the damaging effects of the abuse, once it has ended.

If you suspect that a child or young person you know is being sexually abused, you have a responsibility to talk about it – however awkward or disagreeable that may be. Do seek professional help. If something can be done, you will be protecting not only the young person you know, but possibly many others as well.

If, as an adult, you are sexually abusing a young person you must seek help to stop this happening. Many adults who do have sexual relationships with children tell themselves that it is alright, because the feelings they have are loving feelings, not angry or abusive feelings. This is far from the truth. For a child or young person to be forced to have sex with a trusted adult is one of the most damaging experiences possible, whatever the feelings of the adult may be.

Some adults say that their instincts tell them it is wrong, but that they do not have the strength to stop themselves. Also, adults can easily convince themselves that the young person doesn't mind, or isn't being affected by the experience.

If you are in this position, seek help now. Do not allow your sexual feelings towards the young person to be expressed openly.

If they are being expressed, find a way to stop yourself. You may feel ashamed, or afraid of telling someone. It may well be difficult for you, but if you do have loving feelings towards your child or teenager, then you will want to prevent them from being damaged any further.

Useful organisations

The Children's Legal Centre provides a free and confidential legal advice and information service, covering all aspects of the law affecting children and young people. Their address is: University of Essex, Wivenhoe Park, Colchester, Essex CO4 3SQ. Advice line: 01206 873820.

Citizens Advice Bureau (CAB). Trained workers offer information and advice on a wide range of topics, including legal problems and family and personal difficulties. Anyone can use the CAB, but you may need to make an appointment, or you may be able to call in and wait your turn. Some CABs give advice over the telephone but lines tend to be very busy. To find your nearest CAB look in the telephone book under 'Citizens', or ask at your local library.

9

The parent's role

In this final chapter, I look at some of the issues facing parents as they come to terms with the sexuality of their daughter or son.

The topics I cover include:

The generation gap

Managing conflict between parents

Communication

Recognising problems

Coming to terms with adolescent sexuality

The generation gap

The phrase 'the generation gap' is sometimes used to refer to a difference in values or attitudes between two generations – particularly between teenagers and their parents. It is a phrase frequently used by the media. It is also one that all too easily becomes linked with sensational or frightening ideas, such as 'generations at war' or some similar notion.

In fact research shows that parents and teenagers do have different opinions on some subjects, but not on all. There may be differences about sex, but not about honesty, or politics. Furthermore, having a difference of opinion does not necessarily mean being in conflict, or being at loggerheads. It is possible to agree to differ.

Research also shows that families vary enormously in the extent to which the generations agree or disagree on sexual matters. Parents of young people are more likely to share values, and to have similar opinions about sex, when communication in the family is good. The more discussion there is, and the more respect the generations show for each other, the less the chance of conflict.

Nonetheless, sex is a matter on which parents and teenagers may well disagree. This is not really surprising, given the enormous changes that have occurred over the last 40 years, where sexual behaviour is concerned. The marked changes in society – caused, for example, by the existence of HIV/AIDS, the lessening of censorship, the use of sex as an advertising medium, and the explicit nature of many films, videos and television programmes – have meant that the experiences of one generation are bound to be quite different from the experiences of another. Thus, we cannot really expect people born 30 years apart to have the same values in relation to sexuality:

I think there is a generation gap, full stop. I know even with our youngest son, I can't quite remember what the context was, but he turned round to me and said 'You're so Victorian'. I'd hate to think I was

*Victorian. I think attitudes to things like sex change
so violently even in the space of 10 or 15 years,
parents aren't always going to be able to keep up
with the way the younger generation are thinking
on these things.*

Father of three sons

Particular difficulties arise for young people growing up in
minority ethnic cultures. Thus, it may well be that a
Muslim girl, for example, finds herself torn between two
sets of cultural standards, as well as between two generations. Parents who are Asian, or Turkish, or African, may
face the problem of ensuring that their values – often
rooted in their own religious background – are upheld.
Yet, they and their children may live in a society in
which quite different values are dominant. Differences
between cultures may widen the gap between parents
and teenagers in such circumstances. Parents need to
recognise that the importance of maintaining their
cultural values – especially where sexual behaviour is
concerned – may create particular strains for their sons
and daughters.

If you find that you disagree with your teenager about
sex, try not to let it become a major barrier between you.
Remember:

- young people are entitled to hold different views;
- young people are *likely* to hold different views, given
  their different experiences;
- people with different views do not necessarily need to
  fall out;
- communication is still possible, even if the other
  person has an opinion which is different from your
  own!

Managing conflict between parents

I have talked a lot in this book about the possibility of
disagreement between children and parents. However,
no attention has yet been paid to another sort of conflict
within the family – that between the parents themselves.
Of course, all couples differ in the extent to which they
come into conflict with each other. Some couples hate
arguments, and manage disagreement by allowing one
partner to dominate. Others avoid conflict by each going
their own way. In some families, there may be battles and
arguments over the smallest things, while in others there
may be very little disagreement.

Most couples find one way or another of sorting out
between them how they will manage their children. Of
especial importance here is managing issues which can
cause friction. Most parents learn that it is best to show
a united front. If young people can drive a wedge between
mother and father, playing one off against the other,
relationships in the home are likely to deteriorate. It is
not good for children to have the power to create disagreement between their parents or carers. Many parents find,
however, that their relationship comes under strain when
there are teenagers in the house. The sorts of issues we
have been discussing, such as challenging behaviour, test-
ing the limits, and so on, do push parents to the edge. To
their distress, parents find that they end up rowing with
their partner in a quite unexpected manner. This is especially difficult, since it may be at just this time that
parents most need each other's support.

There are some teenagers who have the capacity, not
just to wind adults up, but to create tensions between their
parents too. If this is happening in your family, try to step
back and look closely at what is going on:

- Have rows between you and your partner increased as a result of your teenager's behaviour?
- If so, ask yourself what the arguments are about?
- Try to see the situation from the perspective of an outsider. This may help you realise how much you are being affected by the teenager's behaviour.
- If necessary, talk to a trusted friend. This may assist you to see things in a different light.
- Find a way to talk to your partner quietly and calmly, preferably away from home. An evening out, or a short holiday, may be a good time to do this.
- Your teenager may be getting a buzz from seeing you at sixes and sevens. Don't let this happen. Re-mind yourself that your teenager needs their parents to be in agreement, not in conflict.

Communication

I have referred a number of times throughout this book to the importance of communication. Yet communication on the topic of sexuality remains a difficult area for parents and carers, so let us look in this final chapter at some of the obstacles, and consider what can be done.

Obstacle 1: 'I am too embarrassed to talk about this'

Many people do feel embarrassed. You are not unusual. Why not start by letting your teenager know that you think it is important to talk, but that you feel embarrassed to do so? To acknowledge this may be helpful to both of you, and bring you close enough to start the process of sharing your views.

Obstacle 2: 'My teenager won't tell me what he/she is doing'

Many parents get discouraged or upset because they feel their teenager is not being open and honest about their emotional life. Parents should not expect teenagers to do this. Because of their uncertainties and anxieties, young people need privacy as far as their relationships are concerned. Communication about sexuality – about contraceptives, sexually transmitted infections and so on – is not the same as sharing every intimate detail.

Obstacle 3: 'I want to talk, but my teenager avoids the subject'

This situation occurs most often because the subject is tackled in the wrong way. Don't force the issue. Choose a moment when your teenager wants to talk. Start by letting them set the agenda. Use a TV programme or another event to open a discussion. Above all, show that you are willing to listen. A good listener is the best communicator.

Obstacle 4: 'I am worried that if we do talk about sex, we will end up in violent disagreement'

This is another common worry. You may find that you and your teenager disagree, but this does not necessarily mean that you will have a violent row. Try to accept each other's differences. If you can do this, you will be accepting that your son or daughter is an individual in their own right.

Obstacle 5: 'I feel completely out of my depth. My teenager probably knows so much more than I do'

There are two ways parents can tackle this. First, they can make sure they are well informed by reading up on the subject, or by watching a video. Your local library will help you. Second, you can be honest with your teenager. If you tell your daughter or son that you are worried about your lack of knowledge, you may find that she/he will be much more open with you too. Having a good discussion may reveal that you have both got things to learn from each other:

> *Well I'd say no matter how hard it is, grit your teeth, giggle, and get it out. Get it out of your mouth, because once you've got it out the first few times it is easier. All I can say really is take a deep breath and have a go. Speaking about it, talking about it. And if you say, I don't know, 'I got this book out of the library because I realised that I didn't know that much and I thought we could learn this together' or whatever, I don't know, but take a deep breath and go for it.*
>
> Mother of two sons

Communication about sex may seem difficult or even impossible to some parents. However, communication is a skill that everyone can learn. You do not have to be clever with words, or have passed lots of exams, to communicate well. Some of the most powerful communication occurs between people without any talking at all. If you want to get through to your teenager, there is a way to do it. The suggestions that I have made will, I hope, help you to do this.

Recognising problems

Some parents or carers may be faced with adolescent behaviour which they do not understand. Others may worry that something the teenager is doing is abnormal, and requires treatment or professional help. For example, you may come home one evening and find your son watching a pornographic video. Alternatively, your daughter may seem to be promiscuous in her sexual relationships. She may be sleeping with a different boy each week, and be proud of it. Perhaps you find girls' clothes in your son's bedroom, and you worry about cross-dressing, or some other unusual behaviour. What do parents do in such circumstances?

This is not the place to discuss problem behaviour in any great detail. Indeed, each problem will probably be unique in its own way. The difficulty for parents is to know if a particular behaviour represents an illness or disturbance, or whether it is within what might be called 'normal limits'. Another issue here is that even if the parents believe the young person's behaviour to be serious enough to require treatment or intervention, the boy or girl may not take the same view.

The first thing to say is that if parents or carers are worried, they should seek professional advice. You may not need to involve your teenager at this stage. An initial discussion with your GP, for example, may reassure you that no further action is needed. Such a consultation may be enough to allow you to see the behaviour in a different light. You may learn that something that you are worried about happens quite often, and that your teenager's behaviour is nothing to be concerned about.

Of course, this first meeting with a professional might have quite a different outcome. It may be that your teenager's behaviour does need some attention. The doctor may persuade you that your teenager does need help. You are then faced with the question of how to involve your daughter or son. However difficult this is, you need to clarify with the young person what they feel about the behaviour. Are they worried themselves? Do they feel they need counselling, or some other form of treatment?

It may be very tricky indeed to discuss this. You will need patience and sensitivity. If you as parents are worried, you can share this concern with your teenager. Try not to be critical, or domineering. If you express your concern in terms of an anxiety about the welfare of your child, you may find it possible to talk with them about the problem.

You need to be prepared for a number of different reactions. Your teenager may be defensive, and deny there is a problem. They may be angry and resentful that you have interfered. However, many young people will be relieved and grateful. All too often adolescents struggle with a deep-seated fear about their strange or eccentric behaviour. They are unable to seek help themselves, but need someone else to acknowledge that they may have a problem. If parents can do this for their daughter or son, they will have done something very important indeed.

Coming to terms with adolescent sexuality

It is no easy task for parents or carers to come to terms with their son's or daughter's sexuality. I have referred to this issue a number of times in the course of this book. When a young person starts having a sexual relationship this is symbolic of maturity. It represents, more clearly than anything else, the fact that the child is now grown up. Of course, one of the dilemmas of today's world is that the

14- or 15-year-old who is sexually active may appear to the parents to be far from grown up.

Nonetheless, sexuality is connected with adulthood. It is also connected with identity and individuality. The teenager who is sexually mature is an individual. She or he is someone who has an intimate relationship with a partner outside the family. She or he is someone whose actions state 'I am now a separate person'. Mothers and fathers have to make a considerable adjustment in order to accept this change in status. Their child is no longer a child. In order to come to terms with this, adults have to let go, and for some this, may be very hard indeed.

To conclude this book I shall turn to three parents – two mothers and a father. What they have to say underlines the advice I have been giving. Their experience will, I hope, prove helpful to all parents and carers stuggling with teenage sexuality.

Accept, but don't always approve

I feel that no matter how much you disapprove of the youngster's sexual attitudes, the chances are that they're gonna do it anyway, and you have to decide whether you are going to bridge that gap and try to understand what they do, or risk them just deceiving you. So you may just have to look away and accept what you don't approve of. And there is a fine line between acceptance and approval.

Play the listening game

A parent plays the part of a shoulder to cry on, support, the knowledge base. It's almost like a waiting role, or a listening game but being aware, and showing the child that you are available for anything, even if it's relatively trivial.

Be willing to cut the cord

There comes a time when we have to let our children go their own way. We have to cut the cord and we have to take them by the hand and say 'Go and get on with it'. We can't do it for them once they've flown the nest, or once they've become sexually active. We cannot take them and give them a condom to wear and say 'Here you are, you've got to use it'. It's up to them.

Good luck.

Useful reading

Parenting Girls by Janet Irwin, Susanna de Vries and Susan Statigos Wilson – Jessica Kingsley (2000). Examines topics ranging from infant development to teenage issues.

How to Talk to Teens about Really Important Things by Charles E. Schaefer, Theresa Foy DiGeronimo – John Wiley & Sons (1999). Offers parents a commonsense approach of what to say to teenagers, and how and when to say it.

Communicating with Your Teenager by Sheila Munro – Piccadilly Press (1998). This book gives parents advice and guidance on how to manage the most common teenage problems.

Teenagers, the Agony, the Ecstasy, the Answers by Aidan MacFarlane and Ann McPherson – Little, Brown and Company (1999). Packed with practical information on how to deal with a wide range of issues.

The Parentalk Guide to the Teenage Years by Steve Chalke – Hodder & Stoughton (1999). Down-to-earth information and advice on how to make the most of all the important stages of your child's growing up.

Useful websites

www.parentalk.co.uk is for parents and lists useful guides, offers advice, news and features about all aspects of parenting.

Index

Also Available in This Series

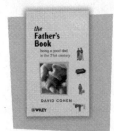

The Father's Book
Being a Good Dad in the 21st Century
0-470-84133-8

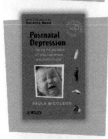

Postnatal Depression
Facing the Paradox of Loss,
Happiness and Motherhood
0-471-48527-6

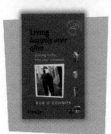

Living Happily Ever After
Putting Reality into Your Romance
0-470-84134-6